the shock factor

Sarah Pickles

The Shock Factor – Sarah's story: beating breast cancer one day at a time

Copyright @2016 Sarah Pickles
www.sarahsstory.co.uk

Sarah Pickles asserts the moral right be identified as the author of this boOK, in accordance with the copyright, designs and patents Act 1988.
All rights reserved. No part of this publication may be reproduced, stored in a retrieval system, or transmitted in any form, or by any means, electronic, mechanical, photocopying, recording or otherwise, without the prior written permission of the publisher.

First published in 2016 by Sarah Pickles
Copyeditor and proof reader: Sian-Elin Flint-Freel
Design and Typesetting: Ellen Parzer
Printed and bound: Create space

ISBN-13: 978-1511954464

All information, methods, techniques, and advice contained within this publication reflect the views and experiences of the author, whose intent is to provide readers with various choices and options. We are all individuals with different beliefs and viewpoints, therefore it is recommended that readers carry out their own research prior to making any such choices. While all attempts have been made to verify the information contained within this book, neither the author nor the publisher assume responsibility for any errors or omissions, or for any actions taken or results experienced by any reader.

DEDICATION

I dedicate this book to my beautiful daughter, Lillie.

Lillie, you have the kindest heart and most beautiful soul. I thank you for being my inspiration throughout my journey. I dedicate this book to you to show you anything is possible, no matter what challenges you face or how tough life gets.

If you have strength, courage and determination and never give up you will find the rainbow. I hope you never have to read this book for anything else other than because you want to understand the experiences we shared as a family and because mummy wrote it!

My one wish from writing my book it is that I can have a positive influence on you and help protect you as you face your own life experiences. I hope I inspire you just like you inspired me.

www.sarahsstory.co.uk

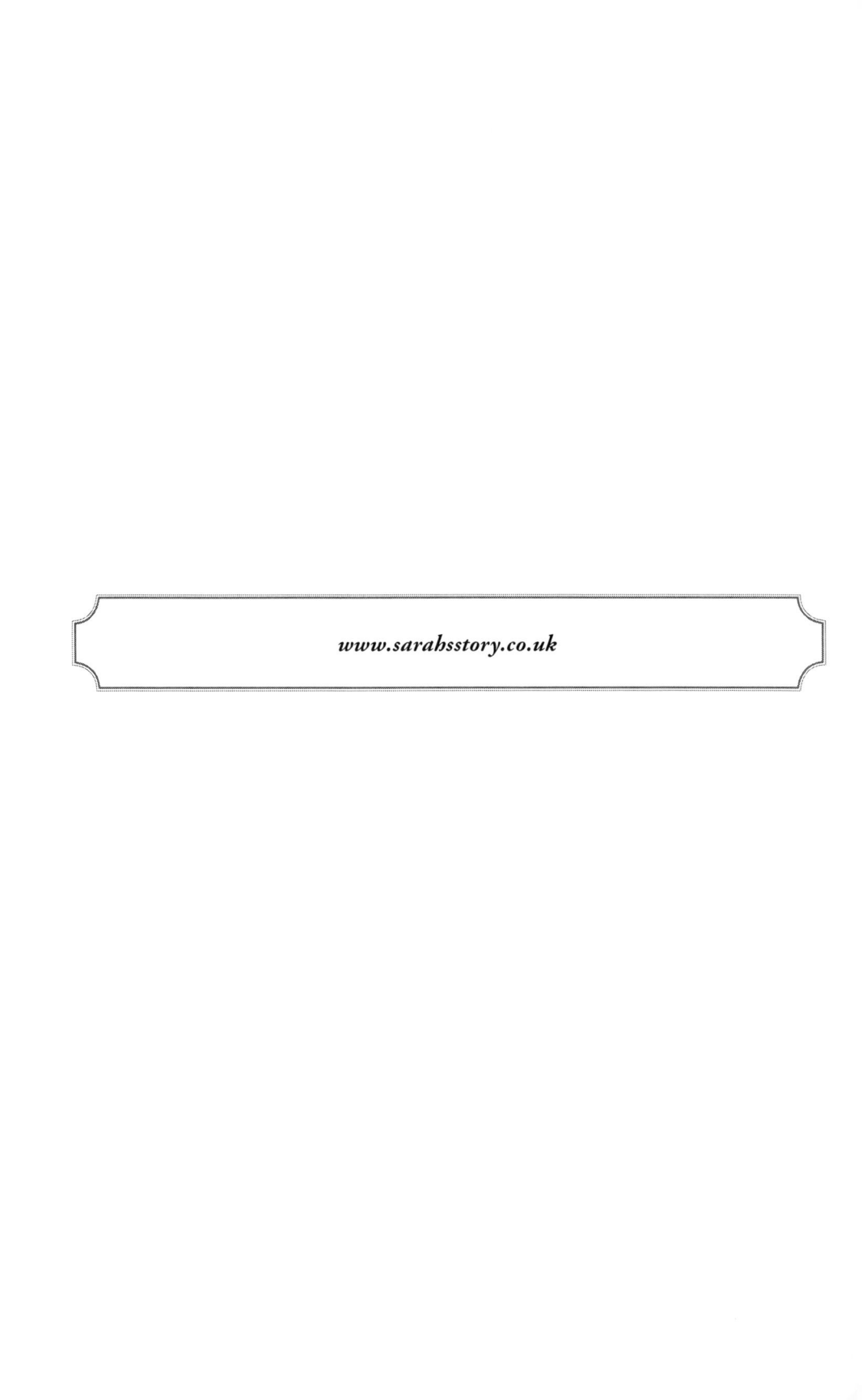

Contents

Chapter One The Shock Factor — 9

Chapter Two How Did I Get To Here? — 12

Chapter Three Breaking The News — 16

Chapter Four Life Changes After Diagnosis — 21

Chapter Five And So It Begins — 28

Chapter Six Hair Today…Gone Tomorrow — 61

Chapter Seven All Things Boobs — 74

Chapter Eight Giving Myself The Best Chance — 98

Chapter Nine Looking Good, Feeling Great — 129

Chapter Ten Planning Ahead — 139

Chapter Eleven One Year On — 148

Afterword — 151

About Sarah — 152

St Luke's Hospice / Macmillan — 153

Useful Links — 154

ACKNOWLEDGMENTS

I would like to say a huge thank you to all my friends and family who have shown kindness and generosity along the way. You have supported me by being there for me when I have needed it most. You have all enriched my life more than you will know. I will be forever grateful for the support that you have shown not only to me but to Dave and Lillie too.

Thank you to all my supporters who have followed my story and shared my page, helping to create awareness. Thanks also to all the beautiful butterflies in my breast cancer group for making the group the success it is, and to a few special ladies who shared some of their own experiences of side effects from chemotherapy in Chapter Five: Joan Hulse, Codilia Garpare, Michelle Mullany, Jayne Andrews, Linda Dolly Edwards and Claire Farnsworth.

A special thank you to Toni Mackenzie (hypnotherapist), Tonje Olsen (physiotherapist), Chris McDermott (energy healer), Fraser White (hypnotherapist), Carol Robinson (personal trainer), St Luke's Hospice, Macmillan, Shine Bright, Navitas Holistic Centre, Leighton Hospital and The Christie hospital for all the support, help, care and kindness you have shown throughout my journey, making it a much more pleasant and enjoyable experience.

Thank you also to my book mentor and editor, Sian-Elin Flint-Freel, for her fantastic support, guidance and patience, and for mentoring me throughout my journey, giving me the confidence to become a writer and an author.

Last but definitely not least, my wonderful husband and my gorgeous daughter, Lillie. You two are the reason I am here today and are my inspiration to write my book. You have both given me the strength and courage to keep focused and to get through my journey. Dave, thank you for being with me every step of the way, always being by my side throughout and for making me laugh with your silly jokes! Thank you for taking on my role as a mummy when I was too poorly to do it. Lillie, thank you for helping to make me feel happy in my darkest hours with your beautiful smile, your humour and your beautiful pictures. I am so proud of the way you helped and looked after me whenever I was feeling poorly. You have so much love, strength, determination and bravery, which made every day of my journey worth fighting for and gave me the courage to never give up.

I will be forever grateful for all your love and support.

CHAPTER ONE

The Shock Factor

The door handle started to turn and I knew this was the moment that could change my life forever. Mr Mahadev appeared with another staff member. He introduced himself and then introduced Sally, a breast care nurse, and sat down beside me. He started to go through my notes: family history, the results of the mammogram and the biopsy. Then he delivered the devastating news...

I'm really sorry but the mammogram has shown two tumours in the left breast.

WOW! My whole stomach exploded; it felt like someone had kicked me. Any emotion I had held back came out all at once. I never thought when I was being screened a few weeks previously that three weeks on I would be given the news that I had breast cancer at 32 years of age.

* * * *

Tuesday, 23rd September, 2014 — the day I was going to find out the results of my ultrasound biopsy.

It was a normal Tuesday morning with the usual hectic routine of getting Lillie ready for school and making breakfast; the only thing that was different was the fact that I would be getting the results of my biopsy. Up until my appointment in the afternoon I didn't think too much about it and carried on my day as normal. The time came to leave for the hospital, so Dave and I set off. I remember the day so clearly; it was beautiful and sunny.

On the journey Dave asked me how I was feeling and my answer was that I was confident and still very much focused on my decision to have a mastectomy to reduce the risks of ever getting breast cancer.

We arrived at the hospital reception in plenty of time and were asked to take a seat. While we were sitting there, Dave and I just chatted about life in general: what we were going to have for tea that night, who was going to cook, and whether Lillie was enjoying her first year of infant school.

Eventually we were called through to the waiting room but had to sit there for another 15 minutes — which felt like a lifetime. At this point my nerves had started to kick in and a feeling of dread crept through my body.

Dave had found a travelling magazine, which had an article about Peru. He was chatting away, showing me the pictures and saying how beautiful it was. I remember wanting to listen but I couldn't because my mind wouldn't focus. I could think of nothing else apart from what was about to happen.

When my name was called we were taken into a side room where we had to wait another five minutes, which again was like a lifetime. By this point my intuition had kicked in and I felt an empty feeling in the pit of my stomach. I already knew.

Then we were given the diagnosis.

Hearing that word tumour made me feel sick inside. I'd met lots of people who have gone through cancer but you never think it's going to happen to you. I looked over at Dave's face, which is normally so happy and smiley, but he was in complete shock and fighting back the tears. His gorgeous smile and the sparkle in his eyes had gone. We listened to the rest of the diagnosis as Dr Mahadev continued, telling me that the tumours were very aggressive and that, because of my age, the cells were growing rapidly so I would need to have chemotherapy and a mastectomy. The tears flooded my face; I had no control over my emotions. All I remember saying was I was going to be brave. Dave and I had so many questions but didn't know where to start. Our whole world had been turned upside down; it was as though we had been transported into a surreal dream.

We arrived home after picking Lillie up from school and the first thing I did was change into my running clothes. I had taken up running at the beginning of the year and had started to run on a regular basis. It helped me to de-stress and gather my thoughts and I had even taken part in a few trail runs. However, this run was different to what I'd experienced before — I was now a runner who had breast cancer.

Despite the emotions that were coursing through me, for the first time in my life I felt totally in control. There and then I made the decision that, no matter what, I would beat breast cancer and would not let it take control of me. *I* would be in control of the cancer and would look for a positive in every aspect of my journey.

CHAPTER TWO

How Did I Get To Here?

It was August 2014 when I decided to go to my doctor to ask for tests which would tell me if I was at a high risk of carrying the breast cancer gene. Breast cancer runs in my family on both sides; my mum and her mum had it, my dad's mum and sister also had it. Unfortunately, my mum's mum died in her fifties as a result of the cancer, but my mum, aunt and other nan have battled through, are out of remission, and are fit and well. As you can imagine, I was concerned about what could be ahead of me. The most important reason for wanting to find out was because of my beautiful daughter, Lillie. I wanted to do everything I could to protect her in the future and I knew that there was a chance she could also be at high risk if I tested positive for the BRCA gene, the one that is linked to breast cancer.

I had enquired about a mammogram in the past but had been told the earliest they would screen me was when I turned 35 (in three years), unless I had the genetic testing done. However, there was a constant nagging feeling in the back of my mind that all was not right. I NEEDED to know. After a visit to my GP, where I expressed my concerns and told her my family history, she referred me to the genetics clinic in Chester.

They responded quickly and called me a few days later to discuss the genetic testing procedure and my family history. As an aside, I had got a bit mixed up with all the facts and told the nurse that my nan was 27 when she died of cancer. In reality, it was my mother who was 27 when my nan died in her fifties. I wonder to this day if things would have been very different if I hadn't made the mistake? Would they have taken my concerns quite so seriously?

After the discussion, the nurse informed me it was not possible for me to be directly tested, as my mum would need to be tested first. Once she had been tested, her blood results would then confirm if she carried *BRCA1* or *BRCA2* — these are human genes that produce tumour suppressor proteins which help repair damaged DNA and, therefore, suppress tumour formation. I could then be tested to see if I also carried the gene. In the meantime, the nurse referred me for a mammogram.

Finally, I felt that things had been set in motion and I was being listened to. I no longer had to think about it constantly. The risk of having breast cancer in the future had been a constant worry and, since hearing about it six years previously, the possibility of being a BRCA carrier had always been on my mind. However, I'd never been worried enough to check my breasts on a regular basis — stupid, I know!

Checking your breasts and recognising the signs

The one thing I must stress is the importance of checking your breasts regularly. Get to know how they look and feel so you will be able to detect any abnormalities early.

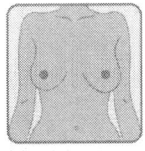
A change in size or shape

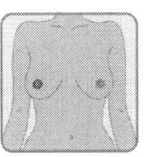
Redness or a rash on the skin and/or around the nipple

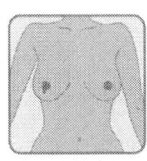
Discharge (liquid) that comes from the nipple without squeezing

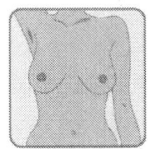
A swelling in your armpit or around your collarbone

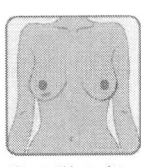
A lump or thickening that feels different from the rest of the breast tissue

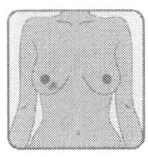
A change in skin texture such as puckering or dimpling (like orange skin)

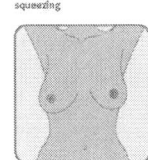
Your nipple becoming inverted (pulled in) or changing its position or shape

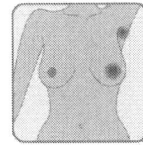
Constant pain in your breast or your armpit

Don't worry if you do spot any irregularities. Most changes to a breast are normal or because of a benign breast condition rather than a sign of breast cancer. Just make sure that see your doctor as soon as you can.

The Shock Factor

My appointment came through the post a few days later. I had made the decision right from the start that if I was a BRCA carrier I was going to have a mastectomy and reconstruction because, even though you may not carry the gene, you can still be at risk of breast cancer, just at a much lower level of risk.

On Monday, 8th September I went for my first ever mammogram. If you have never experienced a mammogram before, you have a treat ahead! The frankly undignified process involves your breast being briefly squeezed between two plates attached to the mammogram machine — an adjustable plastic plate (on top) and a fixed x-ray plate (on the bottom). I was a little bit apprehensive to say the least, as this was my first time.

Monday, 8th September 2014 – Mammogram Day

It's mammogram day! I got to the breast clinic early. The only thing I was interested in was a particularly tasty looking sausage casserole in one of the magazines. That would be perfect for tea! I didn't have long to wait before the nurse took me into another room. Ahead of me were four changing cubicles, just like you'd find in a clothes shop – finally, I felt at home! I took off my top and bra, put on the gown, and waited to be called through to the examination room. The nurse asked me to move forward towards the mammogram machine. I lowered my gown and leant forward as asked. She then placed my boob onto the bottom plate. I had to stop myself from squealing because it was so cold! She then pulled down the adjustable plate and I felt it squashing my boob as it got tighter and tighter. It was a little bit uncomfortable but it only lasted a few seconds, enough time for the x-ray. I was so glad to get my clothes back on.

The nurse told me that I would get a letter in a couple of days and if an abnormality had been detected it would ask me to come back for some further screening. She added that it was nothing to worry about as it was just procedure.

A few days later I received the letter asking me to go back in a week. Because the nurse had told me how the process worked, I didn't feel too concerned at the time. However, a few days later I noticed a small lump on my left breast when I was in the shower. I thought it may have had something to do with the mammogram and that maybe the compression of the plates had caused a blood vessel to swell so thought nothing more of it.

The day of my appointment arrived and I went through the same mammogram procedure as before. As I was having the mammogram, I told the nurse about the small lump I had found. As a result of this, and the fact that they had found two abnormalities in my left breast, the nurse said I would also need an ultrasound scan.

> An ultrasound scan uses high-frequency sound waves to produce an image of the breast tissue.

Once I'd had the ultrasound, the nurse then decided I would need to have a Fine Needle Aspiration (FNA) and core biopsy, which is necessary if a lump or area of concern is found during the breast/underarm examination, mammogram or ultrasound scan.

> A Fine Needle Aspiration (FNA) involves a small sample containing breast cells or breast tissue being taken from the breast to help make a diagnosis, whereas a core biopsy uses a larger needle to obtain a sample and requires a local anesthetic to numb the area. During a core biopsy, a small cut is made in the skin so that samples of tissue can be examined under a microscope in the laboratory.

This is when it hit me that something wasn't right. At no point had I expected to be going through this when I left the house that morning. On my own and completely unprepared, I was still in denial and telling myself that this was just procedure.

As I lay there through the whole process, I was in a bit of a daze, reflecting on the fact that this is what my mum had experienced over a decade earlier. Never did I imagine I would be having it done only 12 years later.

The nurse gave me an appointment to come back for the results the following week. A plaster was put over the insertion area, which I was told had to remain for five days and also not to do any vigorous work or exercise — I've never been good at being told what to do!

The whole experience had been surreal and, although worry had crept in, I knew I had to put it to the back of my mind, carry on, and live life normally until I returned in a week's time, when I would find out if my life would be changing forever.

CHAPTER THREE

Breaking The News

That is how Dave and I ended up in Dr Mahadev's office a week later to hear the devastating words:

I'm really sorry but the mammogram has shown two tumours in the left breast.

That evening, after I had been for my run and finished working in my beauty room, I had to make the phone call to my family and break the upsetting news; the only thing was I had no idea how I was going to tell them. How do you break the news to your family that you have breast cancer?

    I was in shock myself and was still digesting all the information I had been given earlier that day. The memory of receiving the phone call from my mum twelve years previously, telling me she had breast cancer, was still vivid in my mind. I was 22 at the time and remember the moment like it was only yesterday. I was working in my little beauty room when I received the dreaded phone call. Even though you know there is a 50/50 chance of the result going either way, nothing prepares you for the news that you're about to hear. As I listened to my mum delivering the devastating news, my heart broke in two as the tears rolled down my face. It had never crossed my mind that this would happen to my mum. Despite my anguish, I knew it must be ten times worse for her, so I made the decision to take the rest of the afternoon off so I could go home to comfort her and be there as support and help her come to terms with the news.

Little did I know that I would have to relive this nightmare. The only difference this time was that now it was my turn to share this awful news with my mother. Back then, when my mother was diagnosed, breast cancer wasn't heard of as much as it is now. Today, one in eight women get breast cancer and there is much more publicity and information about the disease. However, this didn't make the prospect of telling my family any easier.

Plucking up the courage, I dialled my parents' number. My stomach performed summersaults as the ringtone resonated in my ear and an overwhelming feeling of nausea rose up through my body. I was going to be sick! My mum answered:

Mum: Hello.
Me: Hi Mum.
Mum: Hi Love. How are you?

How often do we answer that question with 'Fine, thanks' or 'Great', not really thinking about our reply? This time was very different. I had thought through every single word. I slowly broke the news '…not great…I got the test results of my biopsy today…' The other side of the phone call was silent as I continued, 'And it's not good news. I've…' I paused, wishing that I didn't have to say the next few words, '… got breast cancer.'

It was the first time I had said those words out loud and I could no longer hold back the tears. I heard the shock in my mum's voice as it slowly started to sink in. To the accompaniment of her quiet sobs, I give her more details about my diagnosis and what treatment I would be having. Desperately I tried to comfort my mother, as well as myself, as I told her how I was going to fight this disease. The last thing you want to hear as a parent is that your child has cancer.

Later that day my dad arrived home from work with no idea his world was about to be turned upside down all over again. My mum has since revealed that when she told him he went into a state of shock, muttering 'not again' as he held his head in his hands and started to cry. This was the fourth time my dad would have had to deal with this disease — his mum and sister have both had breast cancer, along with my mum, and now me, his daughter.

After speaking to my mother, I then called my sister, who was understandably in complete disbelief about the situation and who then had to tell my nieces. Repeating the information a second time was no easier as it felt like I was reliving that moment of diagnosis in Mr Mahadev's office over and over again. I was drained, emotionally and physically.

Once I have finished delivering the devastating blow to my family, I spend the rest of the evening clutched in my husband's arms as we both come to terms with the news.

The next morning I woke up hoping the previous day had all been a terrible nightmare, but unfortunately it wasn't! I had woken up as a different person. I was now a young woman with breast cancer and had no real idea what lay ahead for my future. The only thing I was sure of was that I would stay strong and do everything in my power to beat this horrible illness. There was no way I was going to die; I had too much to live for.

That morning I decided I would still go into college to lecture, as it was important to carry on life as normal as possible until my treatment started. On my way to work the nerves kicked in; I didn't have a clue how I was going to be when I started to break the news to my colleagues. Many of them knew I was going for my diagnosis so I knew they would be desperate to hear the results. How on earth would I react when they asked 'How did it go?'

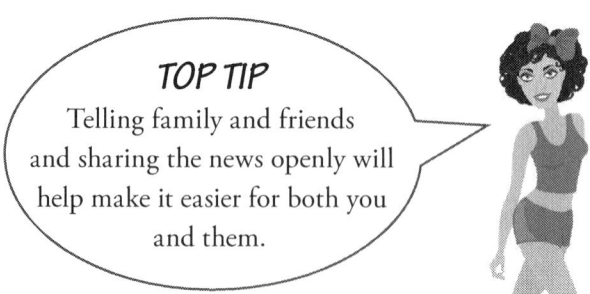

TOP TIP
Telling family and friends and sharing the news openly will help make it easier for both you and them.

However, at no point did it cross my mind that I should keep the news secret from friends, family and colleagues. All along it was my belief that having the information out there in the open made it easier for both them and me. To some degree they would know what to expect and there wouldn't be any awkwardness because someone didn't know how to ask questions about my time off or changes in my appearance. It was also easier for me because people felt they could ask questions. I could speak openly and the support I got was a big…no, a HUGE factor in helping me to succeed.

What to say and what NOT to say to someone with cancer

One thing I noticed through diagnosis was that some people didn't know what to say or they would say things I didn't want to hear. People would get tongue-tied and hesitate, not really knowing what to say. All I wanted to hear was something heartfelt and to feel loved. It's much better to be honest and open.

I wanted to help you out by giving you a list of things NOT to say and a list of NICE things to say if you are ever in this situation. The main thing is don't avoid the person or say nothing! Just to let you know, I didn't have all of these said to me, but I heard a few to say the least!

Things NOT to say to someone with cancer

"I know how you feel."
"Don't worry, things will get better."
"Everything is going to be fine." (You don't know that and it can sound dismissive.)
"Is it terminal?"
"It could be worse, you know."
"All you need to do is think positive."
"I'm sure it's fine. I'm sure it's nothing."
"But you don't look sick."
"Are you better now?"
"But I thought you had chemo and surgery last time. How can it be back?"
"Well at least you will get a new pair of boobs and you don't really need them anyway."
"You look great!" (It's lovely to hear that, but only say it if you truly mean it. On those days when we look like crap, we know when you're not being honest.)

NICE things to say to someone with cancer

"I don't really know what to say but I'm here for you."
"You'll be in my prayers."
"Let me help you with…" i.e. shopping, cooking, etc.
"I will be with you every step of the way."
"Never, never, never give up."
"Do you want me to take you to your appointment?"

> ### *Nice things to DO for someone who has cancer*
>
> Most of all lend a listening ear and just be there. Talk about normal day-to-day life and don't assume they always want to talk about having cancer.
>
> Sometimes a hug is all it takes to make someone feel better.
>
> Sending a card or gift can make a huge difference, especially during treatment when you're feeling low. I remember I was having a really crap day and I decided to pop out to the shops to get out of the house. When I got home my friend had left me a present by the front door. As soon as I saw it I smiled and was immediately filled with happiness.

When I arrived at work I needed to collect some equipment for my class from dispensary. The technician asked me, 'How did yesterday go?' A simple question and one which I had been building myself up to answer during my commute to work but, despite me expecting it, as I started to tell her and said the words 'breast cancer' I broke down. Rather than becoming easier, the more I said the words, the more it felt real. I couldn't believe how much my life had changed in just one day.

As the morning went on, I delivered the news to more of my colleagues. There were lots of tears and they were all in complete shock. Despite the distress, I still believe that going into work was definitely the right decision for me as it helped me come to terms with the reality of having breast cancer. The more I heard myself say the words, the more it started to feel real. In fact, a part of me started to forget what I had felt like before my diagnosis.

From that evening I slowly started to accept that my life was going to change and was feeling strong, focused and ready to take on whatever was going to be happening over the next few months.

CHAPTER FOUR

Life Changes After Diagnosis

My whole life was different after Mr Mahadev's diagnosis. Despite being determined that I was going to be in control and that cancer would not win, managing my own life became increasingly difficult. Although I had every intention of being strong, my vulnerability was never far from the surface because, at the end of the day, I feared for my life. I had every faith in the British National Health Service but there was no guarantee that the treatment was going to work.

It was not long after being given the news that my diary went from being full of business appointments and social meetings with friends to a diary consisting of mainly hospital appointments, the first of which was a pre-op for the lymph node biopsy.

Dr Mahadev didn't think that the cancer had spread to my lymph nodes. However, he couldn't be certain until they had done a sentinel lymph node biopsy, which is basically taking a sample from the first lymph node to which cancer cells are most likely to spread from a primary tumour. (Look at me, knowing all the scientific words!) Since being diagnosed I had become a sponge, absorbing every bit of information to educate myself in what was going to be happening to my body over the next few months. I was constantly asking, 'What is that? How does it work? What is that procedure?'

The lymph node biopsy procedure involves a tiny amount of tracer, either a radioactive tracer (radioisotope) or a blue dye (the one that I had) being injected at the tumour site. The only glimmer of light on this dark day of having a couple of needles puncturing my left breast was that the hospital had arranged for me to get chauffeured to Stoke-on-Trent! This was my time! I felt like such a celebrity. Then the taxi turned up…not quite the limo I was expecting. Good job I'm easily pleased!

Friday, 3rd October, 2014 – Pre-op Lymph Node Biopsy

I set off for the hospital on my lunch break. I had no idea what to expect. Fear set in as the nurse explained she was going to insert two small needles into the breast with the tumours, one of which would be in the areola (the area around the nipple). Squeal!

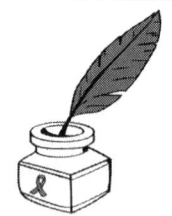

Just a week later, it was time for my MRI Scan.

Friday, 10th October 2014 – MRI Scan

My first ever MRI Scan and I'm not sure what to expect. I am so nervous with the fear of the unknown.

At the MRI scan, after asking some key questions such as DOB, address, and any allergies, the nurse explained the MRI procedure. She then asked me to get changed into a gown…no, sorry, plural…gowns! I had to put on two gowns, one from the front and one from the back, because of the position I'd be in on the platform in the MRI machine.

Now I was getting worried. I'd always had a bit of a phobia about being trapped somewhere where I could not escape (some episodes of 'I'm a Celebrity…Get me Out of Here' freaked me out). It had not really been an issue in my daily life, but this was different.

The nurse placed a cannula in my arm (after two attempts, each time with me getting a little bit more edgy) to feed a dye into my body while I was in the machine.

With as much dignity as I could muster, I climbed onto the plate and positioned myself on all fours whilst attempting to place my boobs in the holders below. Once I was in position, the nurse gave me a pair of industrial headphones to wear, which played music, blocking out the noise of the magnets. In my hand I clenched a rubber button to squeeze in case I had a panic attack — to be honest, there was a high risk of that the way I was feeling!

It was time…they pushed me into the capsule. All I could hear was my own heavy breathing as the door began to close. With a loud, metallic 'clunk' the door slammed and was bolted from the outside. The claustrophobia became overwhelming and I had to try really hard to stop myself from going into a full-blown panic attack. Just in time, the music started. I sighed with relief; the first song was one of my favourites: Ella Henderson – Ghost (you know the one…*I keep going to the river to pray…. la,la,la… the ghost of you eats me away…*something like that, anyway!) It did bring me some comfort as it gave me something else to focus on instead of the ridiculous position I was in! The only problem is every time I hear it now it reminds of this terrifying experience. Despite trying hard to keep control and relax, my mind started to wander. *What if the nurses go off for a coffee break and forget about me…and I'm left in here for hours… or they don't come back at all and I'm left in here with food or water...*

Luckily, none of these fears became reality and eventually I heard a voice through the headphones saying, 'OK Sarah, five minutes left.' It felt like hours had passed but it was 45 minutes in total. Those last five minutes felt like a lifetime. I had already been in this undignified position in my metal cave for 40 minutes; my arms were aching and I had pins and needles in my hands, which then went totally numb.

Eventually I heard the bolt being drawn back, followed by a loud lip-smack of the door's suction. I sighed with relief; it was finally over…until the next appointment.

Wednesday 30th September, 2014 – Lymph node biopsy

I'm not looking forward to today. Having this operation was going to confirm whether the cancer had spread into my lymph nodes.

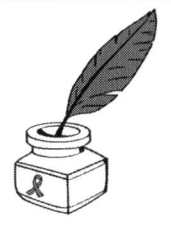

Soon, it was the day of my lymph node biopsy and I was feeling a little bit nervous and scared about it all, as I had no idea what to expect. It also felt very strange, having just been living a normal life one week before, and I was still getting my head around what was actually happening.

It was only a day procedure and a simple operation; they would make a small cut under the arm and at the side of my left breast where the cancer was. They would remove some of the lymph node tissue to test under a microscope, which would show if the cancer had spread.

Before they prepared me for surgery, there were a few forms to fill out. As they asked the questions, I found myself answering but not fully engaging because I was still acclimatising to the 'C' word. It didn't feel real whenever I heard the word come out of my mouth. There was a really nice lady sat next to me as I waited and we soon got chatting, which took my mind of the operation. It is amazing how we are all facing our own battles individually and yet, quite often, walls come tumbling down between patients in a waiting room and the illness that you have in common can make you feel like you have known the stranger next to you for years.

It wasn't long before the porter arrived and I was being escorted in a wheelchair to the pre-op ward. As I arrived I was greeted by some friendly staff who escorted me to a bed where I would have to wait before being taken for surgery. The ward was better than I had imagined; they had recently had a revamp so the décor was very clinical but calming. They had screens put in the ceiling to replicate a skylight, a soothing picture of a beautiful blue sky with white fluffy clouds. To add to this reassuring environment, sounds of nature were played through a sound system to make it feel like you were relaxing outside on a warm summer's day.

I tried to settle down and listen to the beautiful sounds of birds singing but I couldn't stop thinking about what was about to happen. Once I was asleep, I knew it would be OK. However, it had been years since I had experienced a general anaesthetic and the last time I had one I had felt a searing pain up my arm as the drugs entered, before I fell asleep.

Finally it was time for me to go for the operation. As they wheeled me down to the theatre, I gazed at the screens which had also been placed in the corridor ceilings — I can only assume they are there to make patients feel relaxed and to take their mind off what is about to happen. However, as I contemplated the walls painted a very pale sky blue and the blue sky and white fluffy clouds that looked like cotton wools balls on the screens, all I could think of was being in heaven (only, in my perfect heaven, I would be riding a white horse and eating marshmallows…), not necessarily where you want your mind to wander before an operation!

As I lay there, waiting for the anaesthetist to put the cannula in, I was scared and vulnerable and couldn't wait to be asleep to forget everything that was happening just for that moment. Soon I had drifted off into a beautiful, peaceful sleep and before I knew it I had come round from the anaesthetic and was getting excited for my tea and toast!

When I got back to the ward I could smell toast before I even got around the corner. (In my humble opinion, tea and toast is the best part of any operation!) As I waited for it to be brought over my mouth started to water and the more I thought about the delicious melted butter spread over the toast the less control I had over my salivary glands — I had started to drool! The toast arrived and it was delicious…so delicious I had seconds… after all, I thought, I do have cancer!

After a short nap, I was on my way back home, ready for the next appointment.

Monday, 13th October 2014 – Oncology appointment

Today was my first ever visit to Christie's. As soon as we walked through the double doors we were faced with a large waiting area. It was a whole new world full of women who were at different stages in their battle with cancer, some nearing the finish line and others, like me, absolutely terrified and just starting their journey. I have never seen so many women wearing wigs, hats & scarfs in one place. I was an outsider coming into a club where I wasn't a member. Up to today I had been feeling normal and not at all like someone with breast cancer because I hadn't started treatment and still had a full head of hair! Being at Christie's made it real.

My next appointment in my busy diary was at The Christie hospital, Manchester. This was for me to talk to the oncology specialist about the chemotherapy and my treatment options. In one way, I was lucky because part of my treatment would take place at Christie's, which is a cancer specialist hospital with an international reputation. Because of this, I was intrigued about what it was like — and I was not disappointed. Despite what it is there for, the atmosphere was surprisingly welcoming. It even had a relaxation room as an optional waiting room, with couches, a television and computers with Wi-Fi. Dave and I took the opportunity to relax on one of the couches; we giggled about the extreme measures we'd had to go through to spend some quality time together.

My calm mood was broken when my name was called…and eventually disappeared altogether as the information about my diagnosis and my options were delivered in a cold and clinical way, going into graphic detail about what the worst-case scenario could be. I felt sick to my stomach and, although I still didn't completely understand what it actually meant (as most of the information was very scientific), I did understand one thing — I'm going to die.

Of course, that wasn't really the case, but that was all I could think in that moment. The room blurred with my tears as the specialist continued to explain that my cancer was triple negative and, as the tumour cells lacked the necessary receptors, common treatments such as hormone therapy and drugs that target oestrogens, progesterone and HER-2 would be ineffective. Chemotherapy is the only option to treat triple negative breast cancer. My life was being dealt out to me like a pack of playing cards — a pretty bad hand at that.

I suppose for the oncologist it makes sense to be black and white in her delivery because she deals with breast cancer patients on a daily basis, but for me, having just been given the news of my diagnosis, I had not had time to properly digest that I had breast cancer…let alone getting my head around dying! Three weeks ago I was just a normal 32-year-old wife and mummy enjoying life, not thinking for one minute it could change overnight and I would be sat here discussing the devastating side effects of chemo and knowing that this was my only lifeline.

On top of all that, she delivered the news that the MRI had shown there were actually seven tumours in total and that the cancer had spread into my lymph nodes. On a slightly more cheery note my CT was clear and it hadn't spread anywhere else which, looking back, was brilliant news. But at this point it was all too much and as the reality of what was happening hit me I eventually broke down in tears. I couldn't believe this was happening to me — Why me?

Prior to this appointment, my surgeon had explained that having chemo first was the best option as a recent study said that this enabled them to measure more accurately the effects of the drugs on the tumours by MRI scan throughout treatment. By doing it this way round it also reduced the risk of infection, which could happen after the operation and could delay treatment. However, the oncologist felt the best option was for me to have a small operation to have the tumours removed before I started chemo. This confused me completely and I felt torn between two opposing views from two specialists. It was as though she had just chucked a hand grenade into the room, leaving the debris of unanswered questions and confusion, then left!

Dave and I just looked at one another in complete astonishment, wondering what had just happened. We left Christie's feeling very much deflated and emotionally fragile. I cried all the way home, going over everything in my head and trying to make sense of it all.

> ***Here is a list of questions to ask your oncologist before starting chemotherapy.***
>
> - How long will my whole course of chemotherapy take?
> - How many cycles will I have?
> - What hospital will I have my treatment at?
> - How long will each treatment take?
> - What can I do to help myself during treatment to reduce side effects?
> - When will I lose my hair?
> - What are the contact telephone numbers and who do I speak to if I have problems during the night?
> - Will I need any tests before or after chemotherapy?
> - What side effects am I likely to expect?
> - Are there any long-term effects I should know about?

When we collected my daughter on the way home and I saw Lillie's beautiful smile and held her in my arms, any bit of vulnerability disappeared instantly and turned into strength. There was absolutely no way on this earth that I was not going to see my little girl grow up without her mummy. Dying was not an option. I knew I was going to do everything possible to get through the next few months…the first step was a chicken kebab and red wine that night!

CHAPTER FIVE

And So It Begins

The decision was made; I had weighed up the pros and cons of the opposing advice given to me by my oncologist and my surgeon and it was going to be chemotherapy followed by surgery.

> *Friday, 14th November 2014 – My first chemo*
>
> *The day has finally arrived....my first chemo! In a way I'm so happy it is here as the curiosity is starting to play on my mind. I also know the sooner my treatment starts, the quicker it will be over.*

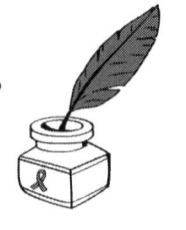

From speaking to the specialists, the Macmillan nurses and remembering what my mother went through, I had a general idea of what to expect as side effects of the chemotherapy drugs:

Side effects of chemotherapy

- Nausea and vomiting;
- Mouth ulcers;
- No taste buds;
- Hair loss;
- Fatigue;
- Infertility; and
- Heart problems.

However, no one really knows how chemotherapy will affect him or her until they experience it. I had most of these symptoms listed above. All I knew was that I was going to do my make-up and wear some heels whenever I could to make myself feel better!

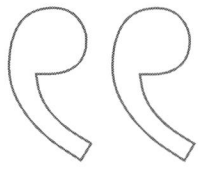

Here are some side effects other ladies have experienced

'Little people with hammers hammering my bones.'

'I felt like I'd got arthritis overnight.'

'I got awful blisters on my nether regions, making it agony to pee.'

'My body was bloated.'

'To this day I can't stand loud noises.'

'When I felt shite all I wanted to do was sleep but the steroids wouldn't let me.'

'The worst pain I have ever known in my joints and muscles.'

'I couldn't use my muscles to sit down or get up off the toilet.'

'I had ulcers so could not eat or drink.'

'A sour taste in my mouth — how I would imagine a fly would taste!'

Rocking my latest hairstyle — the bob — I prepared a rucksack filled with breakfast and lunch items, along with some magazines and my iPad so I could do some writing (from the start, I had decided I was going to write a book about my journey). It felt like I was packing for a fun day out, not a morning of chemo! The surreal part was that I looked and felt so healthy but was actually battling for my life.

Another full waiting room and a sight that was beginning to become very familiar — a range of ladies at varying stages of their own personal journeys, some in headscarves, some in wigs and some wearing hats. Despite this becoming the norm, I tried not to stare, but couldn't help but think, *This will be me in a few weeks.*

Sally, my Macmillan nurse, led us to treatment unit, where we were greeted by all the lovely chemotherapy nurses, including my nurse (Tracy). They couldn't contain their giggles as my glamourous appearance was slightly spoilt by my darling husband accompanying me in his 'winter shorts'! My gaze took in the light and airy room with patio doors looking out onto the beautiful garden, which was still covered in crisp, white snow. *What's all the fuss about?* I thought. *This could be a pleasant morning away from it all!* I had the pick of the room so I decided to go near the window for the view.

Before the treatment started, Tracy talked us through the whole process. We filled in forms and I was given a chemotherapy booklet which had lots of useful information inside, including The Christie's hotline number and a table of a traffic light system to help you identify side effects and how to respond to them. The symptoms were listed under 'red', 'amber' and 'green' alerts, with 'red alert symptoms' resulting in you having to contact The Christie hotline immediately, self-care tips to help deal with 'amber alert symptoms', and 'green alert symptoms' which could be dealt with at home with no further action required. They also provided a handy guide of what to do to reduce the symptoms. This was going to become my diary for the next six months as I filled it in religiously to record the severity of my symptoms.

She then explained how the drugs would be administered, which drugs I would have and the benefits of having them, but more on that later. I had heard some of this previously from my oncologist, however there is so much information being thrown at you and so much to take in that you forget most of it, especially the names of all the drugs — I can't even pronounce them never mind remember them. It's as if you are studying for a course and it's your first day at college — every day!

Once Tracy had explained everything and I had given her the Spanish inquisition, treatment began…

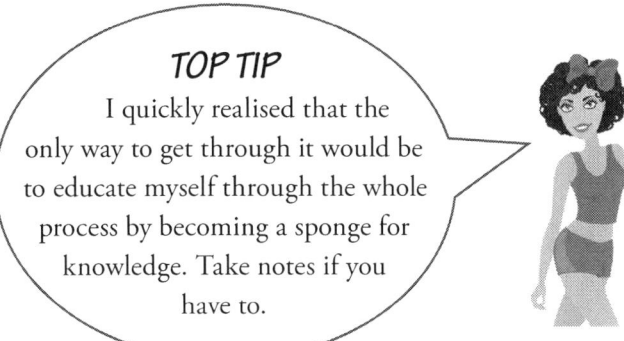

TOP TIP
I quickly realised that the only way to get through it would be to educate myself through the whole process by becoming a sponge for knowledge. Take notes if you have to.

The first part of the process was to place a heat pack on my arm to find some good veins before putting in the cannula — this was the bit I had been dreading the most as I had heard stories of how they sometimes struggle to find veins and may have to cannulate you two or three times. Luckily my veins wanted to join in the party and it went in on the first attempt. All of a sudden I could feel my body start to relax with the relief of that part being over.

Next step, starting to administer the drugs. The drugs I was having at this stage were so aggressive that they had to be administered very carefully by hand to make sure they went into my veins and not my body tissue, where they could cause a lot of damage. The first drug was anti-sickness, followed by the steroids. The nurse pre-warned me that I would experience a strange sensation in my bum for a minute or two — now that was something I had NOT been expecting! I waited in anticipation… here it comes…Wow! I couldn't help but want to clench my bum cheeks together as I experienced the strangest sensation of itching, as though thousands of ants were crawling over my bum — which felt like the longest few minutes of my life! When I clenched my bum cheeks it eased the sensation. Never before had my cheeks had such a workout! Previously, I had never understood why dogs rubbed their bum across the floor but at that moment in time I vowed to have complete empathy with the next dog I saw in this predicament! Unfortunately this wasn't the only time I was going to experience this unusual side effect but I'll tell you about that later. The only benefit of the itchy bum experience was that it took my mind of the next part — the most important part of the process — the cocktail of chemotherapy drugs called FEC.

The drug felt icy cold as it flowed very slowly through my veins and a feeling of exhaustion swept over me (a combination of my adrenaline starting to ease and relief that I had nearly got through my first chemo). As the medicine was being administered I developed an ache in my arm, so when the cannula was finally taken out two-and-a-half hours later it was such a release.

Before we left I was given a goody bag full of drugs — anti-sickness and steroids — to take over the next few days. Weirdly, I felt normal, which was the last thing I was expecting to feel. However, I was also waiting anxiously for the side effects to kick in. When would I have them and how would the treatment affect me?

After leaving the hospital, Dave and I decided to go to Tattenhall village to explore and get some lunch. It was a beautiful winter's day, cold and crisp, but my enjoyment was tainted because I was still in anticipation of something happening. However, all I felt was a little bit tired from all the excitement!

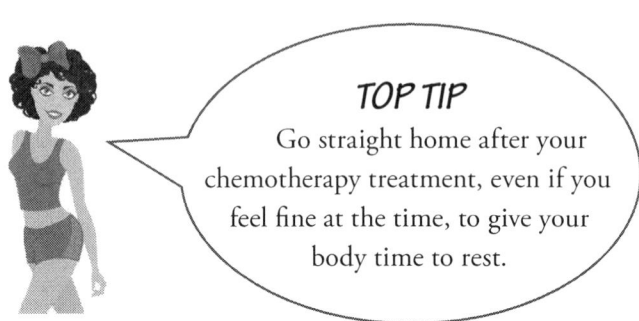

TOP TIP
Go straight home after your chemotherapy treatment, even if you feel fine at the time, to give your body time to rest.

It wasn't until we headed to pick Lillie up that the tiredness really hit me, to such an extent that I had to be dropped off at home for a rest while Dave went to get her from school. Firstly, though, I had to give my mum a call to update her on how my first chemo had gone. Of course, my mum was desperate to know, having been through it herself, but I had to cut the conversation short as my head was pounding and the nausea was creeping in.

After half an hour's nap on the sofa, I woke up feeling absolutely awful. Oh no, it had started! The sickness had really kicked in and my body was a lead weight. I immediately took some nausea tablets from my hospital 'goody bag' and went straight to bed. It was a struggle to take off my clothes and to change into my pyjamas; every movement felt like a major task. I lay there in the darkness wondering what else was to come and how bad it was actually going to get before it got better.

For me, nausea is the worst thing. I would much prefer to be sick, given the choice, and get it over with but the queasiness was pretty much constant for two days after the chemo each time. Sometimes the waves of nausea were so strong that even the powerful anti-sickness drugs couldn't stop them. Despite wanting to throw up so much, it's better not to be sick so that the drugs stay in your body and do their stuff.

Every muscle and bone in my body felt heavy when I woke the next morning after a restless sleep. The nausea, getting up in the middle of the night to take more sickness tablets, as well as feeling the effects of the steroids (that play havoc with your stomach, giving you the sensation of having diarrhoea) had all contributed to a disrupted night. As an added extra, you are pumped with steroids during chemo and have to take additional steroid tablets for two days after. This makes you constipated at the same time as feeling like you have diarrhoea! Feeling like you have diarrhoea and not being able to poo is not a good situation, as you can imagine. Sorry, is that too much information?

After a day in bed, the next morning I woke expecting to feel a little better. However, I felt much worse — my muscles and bones were heavy, my stomach was not great and the nausea was still there; in fact it was even worse than the day before. All of a sudden, the realisation set in as to how my life was about to change, physically and mentally, not only for me but for Dave and Lillie too. The morning after chemo, not only had I woken up in a world of the unknown, but also so had Dave. He had now taken on the role of my carer without being given any textbooks telling him what to do. Although he was extremely sympathetic and capable, he could not feel my pain and discomfort so he was playing a guessing game as he didn't know what to do for the best. He also had to take on my mummy role whenever I wasn't able to do it.

For those two days I stayed in bed, only getting up for the toilet or to stretch my legs by walking tentatively downstairs to get a drink of water. The isolation of being stuck in the bedroom and only being able to spend minimal time with Dave and Lillie was getting to me. I was torn between wanting to spend time with my beautiful daughter and lovely husband and needing to rest. Lillie would pop in to see me at different times throughout the day which helped me to feel hopeful, but she had no idea what was happening, only that mummy had a 'poorly boobie' and was having special medicine to make her better. I didn't even have the energy to get dressed and put on my make-up — which shows how worn out I was.

Waking up the third day after chemo I felt much better than I had done for the last two days. The nausea was nowhere near as bad as it had been. I even felt well enough to get out of bed, get dressed and take on the day — although a little cautiously. I was able to have breakfast — toast and boiled eggs with Dave and Lillie — and although I was feeling lethargic, I was just so happy to be out of bed! Most importantly, finally I was able to poo! I never thought there would be a time that I sat on the toilet celebrating and feeling thankful for being able to take a sh*t! (Sorry Mum!)

Over the next couple of days I had some private teaching work in my diary that I didn't want to cancel unless completely necessary. For me, it was important that I continued to have a normal daily routine whenever possible and to have a reason to get up and have somewhere to be. Of course, everyone is different and it is important that you do what is right for you. What I will say is that, if possible, don't make a decision about work until you have had your first treatment and know how it has affected you. Although teaching helped take my mind off what was happening, it was difficult due to low energy levels, suffering with nausea and having to take my anti-sickness tablets. My students were totally unaware of what I was going through as I had made the decision not to tell them. That is one thing I would have done differently, looking back. By knowing, they would have possibly been more sympathetic and would have a better understanding of why I was dipping in and out of work and why I was less tolerant than usual. By the end of my teaching day I was exhausted. I had completely underestimated the power of chemo.

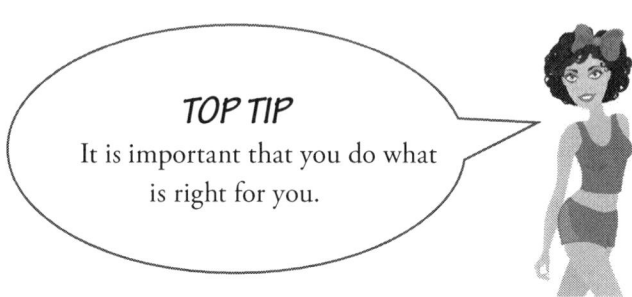

TOP TIP
It is important that you do what is right for you.

Due to the nausea, I had a strong urge for salt and decided I would stop at McDonald's for some chips on my way home from my first day back at work. I was focused more on the salt than the chips, but I didn't think it would be ideal to just eat a salt sachet! The more I thought about the chips, the more my mouth started to water. I couldn't find a McDonald's quick enough! Eventually, after driving three miles out of my way, I saw the golden arches I had been willing to appear. I put in my order:

"Extra-large chips please." My mouth salivated at the thought.

"We don't do extra-large, sorry."

"OK. Two large chips then please." JUST GIVE ME SOME CHIPS!

Not able to wait a minute more, I pulled up in the car park and shovelled them into my mouth like somebody who had not eaten in weeks. As I ate, I could feel the nausea start to subside — it felt so good not to have that sick feeling washing over my body! The only downside was the guilt, as I had started my B-ahead 2 diet (which you will hear more about in Chapter Eight) just before chemo, and chips were definitely not within the diet plan. How was I going to confess this to my dietician?

Despite this little blip, over the next week I stuck to my diet most of the time. However, there were moments in the first week when I would feel so ravenous that I cheated big time but, after that, I followed a strict, healthy diet that didn't consist of two extra-large portions of chips!

For the following two weeks before my next chemo (I had three weeks between treatments), I was back to feeling normal — no nausea, just a bit of tiredness, which didn't have a huge impact on my day. This meant I could now take up running again. Running made me feel better emotionally and physically and gave me time on my own to think. It became my release. That day I only ran three miles (compared with the eight miles I would usually do), but this was enough to fill me up and help me to feel re-energised. From that day on I ran three times week, sometimes four if I could manage it. Exercise played a big part in how I coped during chemo and also in my recovery. It definitely helped towards giving myself the best chance and I will say more about that in Chapter Eight as well.

My second chemo drew closer. It was Monday, a week after having chemo, and things had started to get back to normal. Dave had been in Kilimanjaro leading a group as part of his business and was due back in time to come with me for my next treatment. Lillie and I were in the middle of our usual morning routine; however, this time after breakfast, as we read together I saw loose bits of hair floating onto her book. Puzzled, I reached up only to realise my hair was starting to fall out. I knew this was going to happen within the first three weeks of treatment but I had forgotten about it until that moment. As I pulled my fingers through I couldn't believe the amount of hair that fell to the floor. My eyes filled with tears as Lillie, completely unaware as to what was happening, finished reading the page. When Lillie went upstairs to get dressed, I couldn't resist leaning over the sink and running my fingers through my hair, pulling out all the loose strands and watching as they accumulated on the white porcelain. I was lost in the moment when, all of a sudden, I realised the time. We had to get a move-on. As I prepared Lillie for school, half-listening to her excited chatter about the day ahead, all I could think about was that in a few days all my hair would be gone — it was only going to get worse before it got better.

It was chemo day again — this time being very different to the last. We took minimal stuff and the excitement of that first time had worn off. Instead, there was the anxiety and the expectation of now knowing what was going to happen and the aftermath it left for the next few days. What would the side effects be this time?

As the tomato-red drug, FEC, trickled into my body, I struggled not to think about what it was doing and, instead, tried to relax. (As an aside, the interesting thing about FEC is that when you go for a wee afterwards it would be bright red at first but then would start to run clear. Psychologically you convince yourself that the drugs are no longer in your body.)

Friday, 5th December 2014

This time, for the first time, I actually feel like I have cancer. Most of my beautiful hair has now gone and I am wearing my wig. My nausea kicked in much earlier and happened in the middle of my treatment. I feel so tired. My energy levels have taken a big dip since the first chemo.

Because of what happened last time, we decided to go straight home after the treatment. It wasn't long before I had to take myself upstairs to my bed, where I would be spending the next few days. What made the situation worse was that my first half (three sessions) of my treatment was on a Friday, which meant I would be in bed sick on a weekend, when I would normally be spending time with Dave and Lillie doing family stuff and having fun. I found it very hard coping with the nausea as well as trying to keep my morale strong. My mind ran away with me. This was only my second treatment. How was I ever going to get through the next few months? How did this happen? How can you be living and loving life one minute, then the next your whole world is torn apart as you are struck by a killer disease, wondering what the future holds and hoping you will make it to your next birthday?

I struggled with eating this time round; the most I could manage was a piece of wholemeal toast with a scraping of butter. However, three days later the nausea had subsided and what remained was made bearable with the anti-sickness tablets. I always looked forward to day three because I knew I could get out of bed and I didn't have to take any more of those horrible steroids (which meant I could get a decent night's sleep); but the best thing was that I could poo! Yes, we are on my favourite subject again!

The first thing I would do on a Tuesday morning after Friday's treatment (don't worry, I'm not still on my favourite subject!), even if I didn't feel like it, would be to get dressed and put on my make-up to help myself feel better. I suppose it was also a way of me taking control and showing cancer who was boss! The good thing about the three-weekly treatments was that by week two I was feeling a lot more human and was able to go about day-to-day life. Of course, I still felt tired and there were a few embarrassing issues to contend with…for example, snot leakage!

Let me explain… By now I had pretty much lost my hair everywhere — including my nose hair. The only hair remaining were my eyelashes and eyebrows. I never really knew the purpose for having hair in your nose until this point. If you have never thought about it, let me educate you — it is there to stop bodily fluids from falling out! This happened a few times and was a common side effect of the drug. Sometimes I wouldn't even have time to get a tissue because it wouldn't trickle as it does for normal people with hairs to hang on to, the liquid would literally just fall out of my nose. Once, I was preparing some spinach ready to wash for dinner when, the next thing, some fluid dripped onto a spinach leaf. I couldn't believe it! I was nearly sick and felt so embarrassed, even though I was my own. Thankfully no one was coming for dinner! From then on I had packets of tissues everywhere, ready for any unexpected mishaps! But don't worry if you have had a recent dinner invite from me, my nose is back to its lovely hairy self now so there is no risk of any additional seasoning!

Even though I was having chemo, I still did some teaching to keep my mind active and to give myself a reason to get up and get dressed on days when I didn't feel like it. I also ran as much as possible because, as I said earlier, it helped me not only physically but also mentally. To keep my enthusiasm high and to have something to focus on I set myself a challenge to run three miles every day until my next chemotherapy treatment. To help me stick to it, I posted on my breast cancer Facebook page and gave regular updates when I had completed my three miles each day. It wasn't easy as my fitness levels had definitely been affected by all the drugs and some days would be more difficult than others. It all depended on what else I had done that day because my body tired much more easily. However, the exhilaration I felt once I had done it made it all worthwhile.

My third chemo was going to be on New Year's Eve. In a way I was glad I was able to celebrate most of Christmas feeling well and not spending it in bed. However, this then meant I would be spending New Year's Eve in bed instead. What a difference a year makes! When I was celebrating Christmas 2013 I had no idea I would be battling breast cancer twelve months later.

Christmas day was lovely but inevitably felt a little bit out of the norm due to the circumstances. Thankfully, as I say, my three-weekly treatment fell perfectly, which meant I was feeling great with no sickness or nausea the two weeks leading up to the big day. I absolutely love Christmas and always like to make it extra special, even more so since having Lillie. This year we started putting some of the decorations up in the middle of November because we didn't know how I was going to be feeling nearer the time. I even did my Christmas shopping early for the first time ever! I made the decision that this year it was important to spend Christmas day with my family, given the situation.

Dave, Lillie and I had a lovely, relaxing morning at home, unwrapping our presents together before heading off to my parents in the afternoon. One of the big things I noticed that was hugely different this Christmas day was that I didn't have to start getting ready ridiculously early because I had no hair to style! Normally I would have curled my hair, putting it in heated rollers for a few hours because it was so long. This year, my wig was pre-styled and ready to go! It was important for me to look and feel good, so I opted for my sparkly Christmas jumper with a black skirt and a pair of sexy stilettos — I felt fabulous!

Christmas Day, Thursday 25th December 2014

Yay! It's Christmas! Had the most amazing day. Christmas lunch was delicious and it was lovely spending time with my family. But there were moments when I felt like I was outside, looking in. From the outside, this looked a wonderful, happy family occasion (and it was) but I also caught myself wondering what the scene would be like next year...and would I be in it?

However, these moments of darkness didn't spoil my day. By the evening I felt quite exhausted but that was because I'd had such a wonderful time.

After a few days at home I started to prepare myself for chemo by cleaning the house, doing all the washing and the food shopping. This became a bit of a routine, as I knew that in a few days' time I wouldn't be in any fit state to do anything. Thankfully this was going to be the last FEC. I was so happy this part of the treatment was coming to an end; I hated the way it made my feel.

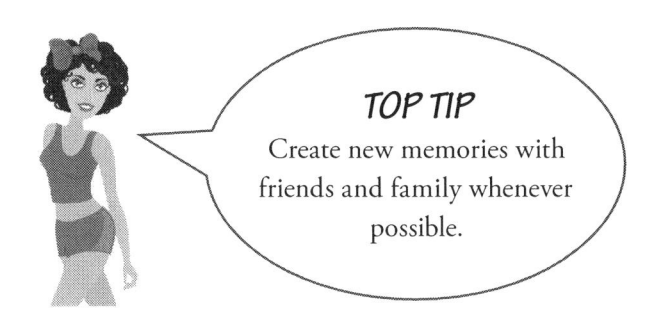

> **TOP TIP**
> Create new memories with friends and family whenever possible.

It was important to me to create new memories with friends and family as much as I could. Before my next chemo we had arranged to go to walking up the beautiful hills of Church Stretton with friends.

Sunday, 28th December 2014

We had such a lovely time today and the scenery was stunning. The further we got up into the hills, the green fields disappeared into the distance and we were in an exciting landscape of glistening white snow. I was energised. After a couple of hours walking and a few snowball fights, we ended the day with some delicious food. At times like these it is hard to believe I am actually battling with breast cancer, feeling as well as I do tonight.

As I got closer to chemo day I started to think about it more and more. Dave, Lillie and I had arranged to go skiing at 'Chill Factore' (an indoor skiing and snowboarding slope) with friends the evening before the next treatment. Spending time with family and friends just before chemo helped take my mind off what was happening and made me feel normal for a few hours.

The day I had been anxiously waiting for — chemo day number three! I was feeling focused but very tired after the excitement of Christmas — it had definitely taken its toll but it was worth it because I had enjoyed every second of it.

One thing that I noticed with my chemotherapy this time was feeling nausea before the treatment had even started. Physiologically I started to think about the drugs going into my body and the effects I would feel later. It didn't go away and continued throughout the treatment, making me feel awful. Being nauseous can be just one of the side effects that can happen whilst chemotherapy is being given.

> *Here are some other side effects that can occur during chemo:*
> - A rash;
> - Feeling itchy;
> - Flushed or short of breath;
> - Swelling of your face or lips;
> - Feeling dizzy;
> - Having pain in your tummy, back or chest; and
> - Feeling unwell.

New Year's Eve, 31st December 2014

As I was being prepared for my New Year's champers (a cocktail of chemo drugs), I was feeling very nauseous. They'd given me a strong anti-sickness tablet to take before treatment but it didn't seem to have had an effect. Normally I have my chemo on a Friday but today I had it on a Wednesday, which meant I could have a reflexology treatment – Woohoo! A New Year's Eve treat!

Dave cooked Lillie and me a delicious supper of homemade lean steak burgers from the farm shop and some broccoli. It was such a perfect moment: the highlight of my New Year's Eve was the three of us sitting in bed together. I couldn't eat much as the sickness started to set in again. Despite my feeling of true happiness as I lay in bed, it filled me with so much sadness that once Dave had put Lillie to bed he would be sat all alone on New Year's Eve – this is the first year since we met that we haven't celebrated together.

One of my foremost memories of that New Year's Eve is waking up a few hours later to the sound of fireworks so loud it felt as though they were right above the bedroom. I remember being so exhausted and sick that I didn't even have the energy to get out of bed and look at them through the window.

The first morning of 2015 felt strange. I had started my journey in 2014 but the real challenge was about to start. Waking up on New Year's Day with the symptoms of a very bad hangover, but not having actually consumed any alcohol the night before, felt weird. I pretty much knew what my New Year's Day would consist of — staying in bed all day — however, I didn't feel completely alone as I knew a majority of the population would be in bed too! Lying in bed I reflected on the last few months of 2014, about how different life had become and how I had changed as a person and become much stronger since my diagnosis. Today I was feeling a little sicker than normal. However, Dave had made a delicious homemade tomato soup and, as the divine aroma drifted upstairs, I couldn't wait to try it. Unfortunately I only managed three mouthfuls before my nausea got so bad that the chances of me being physically sick were very high. Oh no, it was going to happen! I attempted to run as quickly as I could to the bathroom — luckily we have an en suite in the bedroom so I didn't have run too far. It was like a scene from 'The Exorcist'! This was the first time I had been physically sick since treatment started and, although feeling better for being sick, a part of me was worried about depositing some of the drugs down the toilet, thereby reducing their effectiveness.

That experience made me experiment with what types of food were best for me when I was feeling nauseous without having a recurrence of the tomato soup disaster. I found the only thing I could stomach and that seemed to help with the sickness was a boiled egg with a slice of wholemeal toast.

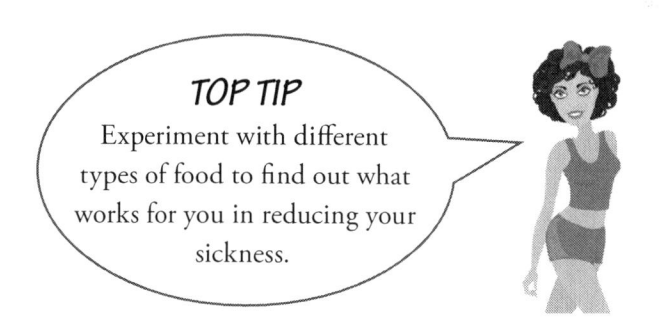

> **TOP TIP**
> Experiment with different types of food to find out what works for you in reducing your sickness.

The next day I woke up feeling moderately well, with just a small amount of nausea (easily controlled with the good ol' anti–sickness tablets) and tiredness. I was very excited as my birthday was on Friday and the way the chemo dates had fallen meant I would be feeling well for my birthday celebrations — every cloud and all that jazz!

I was also celebrating that I was halfway through treatment. The next step was a weekly chemo for nine weeks. The drug I would be having was called Paclitaxel, a less aggressive drug and one that was given in smaller doses. Alongside the Paclitaxel I was going to be having a drug called Carboplatin, a new drug for patients with a triple negative cancer, believed to prevent the cancer from returning over a much longer time period. However, due to the extent of the possible side effects, they wanted to try it on younger patients first to see how they responded. I was willing to do anything and everything to give me a better chance of survival and live a longer life so was happy to be part of the study. This meant my treatment plan would now have to change and could result in more extensive repercussions.

I decided to forget about chemo until after my birthday at the beginning of January (the 8th, in case you want to send a card next year). However, it was much easier said than done. When I woke up on the morning of my birthday it felt very different to every other year — I was bald for a start! Emotionally I didn't feel present and was distracted by what was still to come from the second half of chemo. It was surreal and definitely NOT what I wished for the year before when I blew out the candles on my birthday cake. I didn't want anything too extravagant for my birthday celebrations; I wanted to keep it low key. This year it didn't feel that important, which is not like me at all — in our house we usually have a birthday week! Even though Dave knew how I was feeling, it was important to him to make me feel extra special because of what was happening so he showered me with LOTS of flowers, champagne and chocolates and cooked me a delicious three-course meal — it was perfect and I was able to eat my meal in my onesie with no make-up on and no wig! After the meal I chilled out in the lounge in front of the fire — I felt the cold a lot whilst having chemo…whenever I wasn't having a hot flush!

It was leading up to my fourth chemotherapy treatment and I was starting to worry about this extra drug I was having (Carboplatin). Although it was a new drug that was being trialled, they had already linked it to a range of possible side effects including nausea and vomiting, problems with liver function, tiredness, stomach pain, body aches, diarrhoea, constipation, risk of infection due to a drop in white blood cells making it harder to fight infection, breathlessness, anaemia, a high risk of infertility, and hair loss. (Just a few possible side effects then!) Although Paclitaxel (the drug I had up to then and would continue to have) had its side effects, they were minimal and I knew what to expect; having Paclitaxel felt like an old friend who could get on your nerves, whereas I just didn't know what the impact of Carboplatin would be on my body. I had already lost hair from everywhere apart from my eyebrows and eyelashes due to my treatment so far, so it was highly likely that this new combination of drugs would end up with me losing those last remnants of hair too over the coming weeks. Cancer would have completely stripped me of my identity, causing more heartache and upset.

There were two options with the new drug: I could have small doses of Carboplatin incorporated into my Paclitaxel dose (to minimise the side effects) or have a big dose of Carboplatin every third week. At this point I still had no idea how my body was going to respond to this new intense drug or to what extent my body was going to suffer. However I didn't want to take the risk of being unwell every week for the next six weeks and decided I could cope better mentally by being severely unwell every third week.

> *Thursday 15th January 2015 – Chemo Day number 4*
>
> *My first appointment with my oncologist to discuss the second half of treatment and to see how I have dealt with everything so far. Once the decision had been made about the Carboplatin, my oncologist informed me it would be starting today! All of a sudden I felt sick! Not only was it the uncertainty about the side effects of having this drug, but it also meant I would be having another round of steroids (itchy bum alert!) Whilst waiting for treatment, I started to prepare myself mentally, accepting that I would be out of action but to what extent I don't know. On a positive note, at least I would only have two more left after this one – although I have to survive this one first!*

This was my first treatment at The Christie Hospital in Manchester; the chemotherapy unit was much bigger than the Macmillan unit at Leighton and worked at a much quicker pace to get through all the patients.

As we got to the treatment unit, I gazed with astonishment at how many people — men and women, young and old — were being treated for cancer. There were so many treatment areas and the waiting room was full of patients still waiting to have treatments done. Each of these patients was on their own journeys and facing their own battles. Their friends and families had to deal with the same (and more) challenges that we were tackling. Cancer affects so many lives.

My chemotherapy nurse greeted us with a big smile before escorting us to the treatment cubicle. Each patient had their own separate compartment with walls either side but each was open at the front, allowing you to see the person opposite. I remember thinking that this was nice for anyone who didn't have someone with them so they could chat to someone else — although sometimes you didn't want to talk, you just wanted to rest. I noticed some of the cubicles had reclining chairs and others just had normal chairs with high backs, so I guessed it was just pot luck as to what was available at the time of your treatment.

That day I struck lucky as I got a reclining chair! My chemo nurse introduced herself as Sian as I got myself comfortable in my chair. Sian was so funny and kept me amused — which is always a plus during treatment! She explained what was going to happen, before going off to warm up a heat pack for my arm. This was done at the beginning of every treatment to entice the veins — similar to fishing, I suppose; the heat was the bait and the veins would feel the warmth and congregate towards it, the one unlucky vein (if they got it first time) got the cannula! This was the bit I always dreaded the most. In anticipation of what was to come, my body would stiffen and I would be petrified about whether the needle would go in first time.

Before Sian had even opened her mouth, I knew the two familiar words that were about to roll off her tongue: 'Sharp scratch,' as she inserted the needle into my vein. As I held on to Dave's hand, squeezing it tightly and cutting off his blood supply, the cannula was inserted and my body started to soften as the first drug was administered.

The first was always the anti–sickness drug, swiftly followed by the itchy bum experience (steroids). This delightful(!) symptom only ever lasted for a minute but it felt more like ten! The nurse administered these drugs, whereas the rest were then given to me via a drip.

Carboplatin took an hour to enter my bloodstream and was followed by a 15-minute saline flush. Then Paclitaxel took half an hour, finished by another 15-minute flush of saline.

Whilst having treatment I drank a lot water to help stop me from feeling sick; it also helped to flush the drugs around my body. Sometimes I could taste the chemicals so would have to eat chewing gum or suck mints.

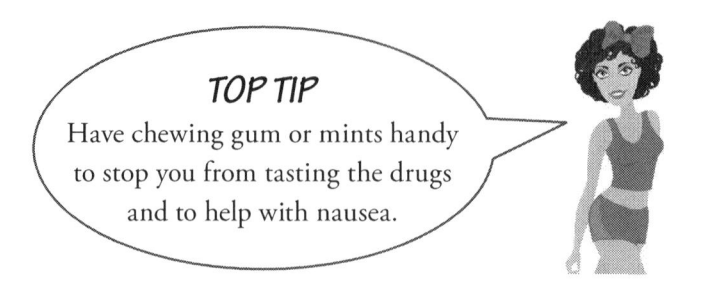

> **TOP TIP**
> Have chewing gum or mints handy to stop you from tasting the drugs and to help with nausea.

After drinking so much water, I needed to go to the toilet and decided to take a different route, going on a little tour. I couldn't believe there was another section of the ward that I hadn't seen, with more treatment bays and yet more people. My heart filled with an overwhelming sadness and my eyes started to fill up, seeing so many fragile and vulnerable people fighting for their lives.

By the time I got back from the toilet, my machine was bleeping, which meant treatment was over. (Time generally passed quickly when I had my chemo buddy, Dave, by my side as he always kept me entertained!) Once the cannula was removed, I was given my goody bag of drugs for the next few days, including some injections called G-CSF (granulocyte-colony stimulating factor). This helps your body to make more white blood cells. Having chemotherapy for cancer can affect your bone marrow, reducing your ability to make new white blood cells. I had to inject myself into my tummy each day. G-CSF can also have some side effects, such as bone pain, itchy skin, or a fever.

That evening I waited with anticipation to feel sickness on a much higher scale than before, expecting to be in bed for a few hours. However, this was not the case. I felt very tired with a little bit of nausea but it was manageable.

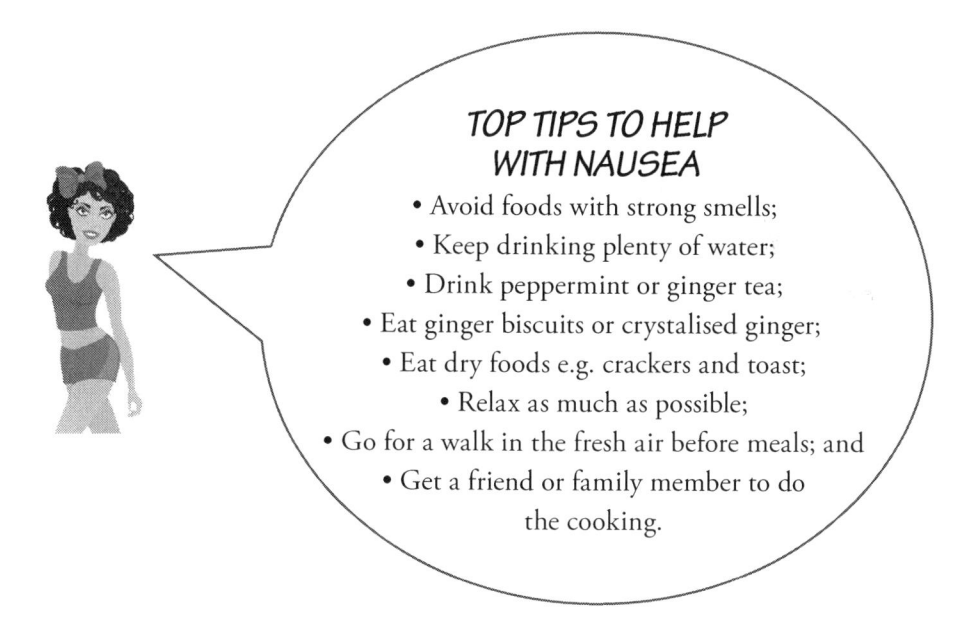

TOP TIPS TO HELP WITH NAUSEA
- Avoid foods with strong smells;
- Keep drinking plenty of water;
- Drink peppermint or ginger tea;
- Eat ginger biscuits or crystalised ginger;
- Eat dry foods e.g. crackers and toast;
- Relax as much as possible;
- Go for a walk in the fresh air before meals; and
- Get a friend or family member to do the cooking.

As the days went by, the side effects became stronger; more nausea along with aches and pains in my joints combined with soreness in my muscles from the injections. I also suffered with constipation from the steroids, which caused some abdominal pain; however, this only lasted for a couple of days.

It wasn't long before I was back at Christie's for my second dose of Paclitaxel. I was much more relaxed this time as I knew it was a shorter treatment and there would be no nausea. After this, I wouldn't have to see the oncologist for another two weeks. The other benefit was I could start going to my local hospital, Leighton, to have my bloods done and this would be the day before chemo. This was a great advantage as previously my bloods would be done on the day of chemo and often meant I had to wait around for hours for results, sometimes delaying my treatment.

Christie's is one of the biggest cancer hospitals in the country and this meant that they were prepared for your every need. If they were running behind, Dave and I could sit in the relaxation room until they were ready, when they would call my mobile. However, before we went to the relaxation room, we always had to go to Starbucks — yes, Christie's has a Starbucks café! I love Starbucks and had decided it was going to my weekly treat whilst having chemo.

As well as the reclining chairs in the treatment rooms, they also had beds so, whenever there was a bed free, I had my treatment done there instead. Also, whenever possible I asked for a spot by the window as it made such a difference to see daylight and feel the freshness from the cold glass during treatment.

Thursday, 29th January 2015 – Chemo number 5

When we got home I felt a little exhausted so had a little sleep on the couch. I woke up having slept peacefully for a couple hours and decided I wanted to go for a run... Dave just looked at me as if I had gone mad and asked if I thought it was a good idea. I felt fine after chemo and rested after my sleep and it was just something I wanted to do. I got changed and off I went on my usual route with my woolly hat on to keep my head warm. It felt so good to be outside in the fresh air and I could feel the sharpness from the freezing cold on my skin as I ran against the wind. My pace wasn't my usual pace but I couldn't have gone any faster. I had planned to only do a mile and a half; two and a half miles later I arrived home. As Dave opened the door I could see the relief in his face. The run has totally re-energised me both physically and mentally and I feel brilliant.

That week I started to feel quite exhausted and was experiencing breathlessness.

I had also noticed my eyebrows and eyelashes were falling out. My poor body not having much time to heal in-between each Thursday's treatment was starting to take its toll.

Every Wednesday before chemo I would have to go to phlebotomy for my bloods to be done. Each week I was given a blood form from Macmillan and would hand this green sheet in to the person on the reception desk. As soon as they realised you were a cancer patient you got special treatment — a bit like a VIP! No matter how full the waiting room was, you got to the front of the queue — the green form was a bit like a queue jump ticket you get at an amusement park. However, you do receive some very, shall we say, interesting looks and sometimes abuse from the other patients waiting to be seen, until you casually tell them that you've got cancer and then they generally want the ground to swallow them up! However, there are a few that couldn't care less what you've got. I once had an interesting experience whilst waiting to have my bloods taken. As I received my green queue jump ticket and took my place at the front of the line, I heard a couple of ladies huffing and puffing, telling me I needed to collect a ticket. The look on their faces when I politely explained that having cancer gets you a VIP ticket was priceless!

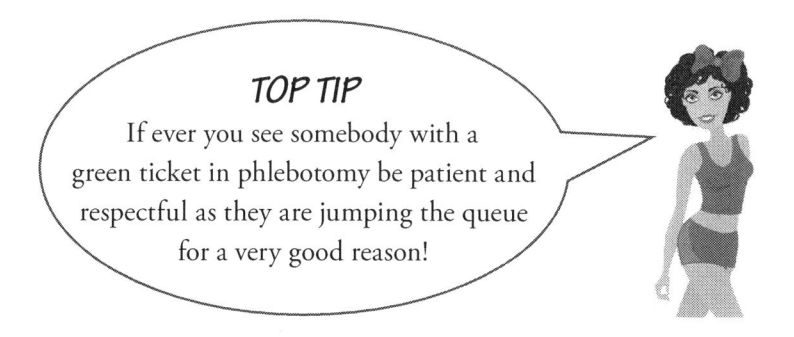

> **TOP TIP**
> If ever you see somebody with a green ticket in phlebotomy be patient and respectful as they are jumping the queue for a very good reason!

I felt looked after each time I went to phlebotomy, which probably sounds really strange…but it's because they are so good at what they do and make the whole experience painless, even pleasurable compared to having a cannula put in! Not once in all the times I've been have they had problems finding a vein and drawing blood. (Once, I asked how many patients they saw in one day. Each nurse can see up to 100 patients, so it's no wonder they are good at it!) Every afternoon after phlebotomy I would receive a call letting me know whether my bloods were OK and, in the two weeks since I had started my weekly chemo, my bloods had been great. However, one of the possible side effects of Carboplatin eventually kicked in.

Wednesday 4th February 2015

Today I had my blood taken by the man who's taken my bloods before and he's always very chatty and always seems pleased to see me. A few hours later I received a call from Sally to tell me that my blood count was low and that chemo will not go ahead tomorrow. From Friday they want to put me on injections to boost my white blood cells to make sure chemo goes ahead next week. Today I was meant to be having another dose of Carboplatin. I am so frustrated not being able to have it because I'd focused my mind-set on the end date and each treatment meant I was one step closer to it all being over.

The low blood count was one of the possible side effects of the Carboplatin. Despite Sally (my Macmillan nurse) being lovely when she phoned to tell me, it was always a huge disappointment. There was nothing I could do whenever my chemo was cancelled because of my blood results, apart from look forward to a week off and take myself to one of my favourite coffee shops, such as 'The Hollies' down the road, where I spent the day drinking coffee and writing my book. I always had a lovely experience whenever I went there and the members of staff were always very friendly… oh, and they serve great cakes!

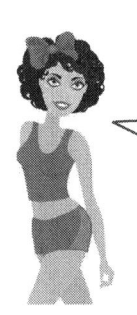

TOP TIP

Try not to get disheartened when you have a setback with treatment. Think of something nice to do with your time, maybe meet with a friend, take yourself somewhere special to read a book, or go shopping and have a nice lunch.

When chemo was postponed, I would have to give myself an injection in my tummy every day from the Saturday until Monday. On Wednesday I would go to phlebotomy to have bloods taken and then wait patiently with everything crossed to hear whether or not I could have chemo that week.

> **Wednesday, 11th February 2015**
>
> I can't believe another week has passed and it's phlebotomy day! When I arrived in reception, the guy who took my bloods last week greeted me. "Hello smiler," he said with a big smile. I blushed and give a little giggle. When I asked him how he was he replied with, "All the better for seeing you with your cheeky little grin." I giggled again before running off with my queue jump ticket…I can still pull, even with cancer! A couple of hours after getting home, my phone rings. It's a private number and I know it is Sally, but for a few seconds I just stare at the phone, letting it ring because I'm too scared to answer it in case it's bad news about my bloods. I finally answer and wait with anticipation until Sally's soft voice eventually tells me my bloods are OK to have chemo!!! I never in my life thought I would get so excited about having treatment. I can't wait to give my chemo buddy the good news.

It was so comforting to know that Christie's were always one step ahead when it came to my treatment, and every time my chemo was postponed I would have an appointment with my oncologist the day of my next treatment. Dr Horsley always put me at ease with her soft Scottish accent; she was attentive, listened to my needs and was always dressed impeccably.

Obviously, with Carboplatin being a new drug, Dr Horsley was keen to know how I felt after the last dose. I'd had aching joints and pain (which resulted in me taking codeine phosphate, as paracetamol wasn't enough to ease it), a bit of nausea and tiredness. She was pleased with how my body had responded and asked if I was still happy with the treatment — to have a big dose every third week. I was. However, due to my bloods being low the week before, she also wanted me to keep having the injections to prevent having to postpone chemo again.

So the treatment continued that day. Once Sian had put in the cannula I could relax. Dave went to get my chemo cap — what I called my cappuccino treat from

Starbucks — with cream and caramel sauce! I even had a foot massage from an adorable holistic therapist called Ann. It was so relaxing I fell asleep — the result of a combination of exhaustion and being treated on a bed. This chemo thing wasn't all that bad!

Each week we would be offered lunch at the hospital. You could choose from a choice of sandwiches, soup, fruit, cheese and crackers. Dave always prepared a packed lunch for us to take in to hospital, which I have to say was much more delicious — but more on my B-Ahead 2 diet in the Chapter Eight.

> *Friday, 13th February 2015*
>
> *This weekend I've taken Dave and Lillie away to Aberdovey in Wales for a Valentine's treat. I hope I'm going to feel OK and not too poorly. When I booked it I'd arranged the timing for when I only had a small dose of chemo but because it got put back a week, it hasn't worked out. It's really important to me to have some time together away from home with no distractions, to completely relax and re-energise as the last few weeks have been a bit challenging. The seaside seemed like the perfect place! When I woke up this morning, my head felt like I had been on the red wine the night before! I had a bit of nausea but nothing I couldn't manage with anti-sickness – nothing was going to stop us from going on our little holiday. We've arrived in Aberdovey and I'm already feeling rested! The journey down was beautiful. We stopped off at a delicious fish & chip shop in Bala and got chips with LOTS of salt and vinegar...they always taste even more delicious after chemo because the steroids make the body crave salts and sugars.*

Over the next couple of days I continued to experience sickness (but controlled it with anti-sickness medication) and felt like I had an extreme hangover, no taste buds and aching as though I'd been beaten with a stick. My muscles were tender from the injections and the ache in my joints (controlled with codeine phosphate) was a constant presence. We continued to enjoy our holiday, even though some days we just stayed in, played board games and watched Disney movies because I was too exhausted to go out. We did manage a day at the seaside, eating ice cream and crabbing, which was great fun, especially when a seagull did the biggest poo on my head! We managed to make the most of our holiday, even with chemo (and the seagull) trying to be a party pooper (literally) and spoil it!

When we got back home on the Tuesday there was a letter from St Mary's, the hospital where I had my genetic testing. My heart sank as I read the letter, convinced it was going to confirm I was a BRCA carrier, meaning Lillie would be at high risk of getting breast cancer in the future. As I continued to read I couldn't believe it… I didn't have the gene! I was totally taken aback by the results because I was convinced I had it due to my strong family history of cancer. This was fantastic news for Lillie because it meant she wasn't a high-risk. I felt relieved and happy knowing my beautiful little girl was safe. However, it left me feeling confused and frustrated because for all this time I had thought my cancer was because I was a BRCA carrier and had come to accept this was the case.

All of a sudden it was just down to unfortunate circumstances and I have no definite idea what actually caused it. This then made me question everything; I wondered whether there are still genes that I may have which would indicate that I am a carrier — but these genes are not yet identified. There must be some connection having such a strong family history?

It's scary to think they won't screen you early unless you have the gene. What do they measure this against? I didn't have the gene yet I had breast cancer at 32. What if the nurse I spoke with initially didn't send me for a mammogram, making me wait until my mum was tested? What if her test results showed up negative? Would they have felt it less important to screen because I wasn't a high risk? If I hadn't followed my gut instinct to contact the doctor in the first place about genetic testing and if the nurse hadn't sent me for a mammogram, what would my situation be now? Even though I wasn't carrier of BRCA, did it actually mean Lillie was a low risk?

This is why it is so important for men and women to check for signs of breast cancer on a regular basis. I never knew what signs to look out for and want to share them with you in the hope that it can help you and others.

When you check your breasts regularly, get used to how they look and feel normally so you can notice anything out of the ordinary. Using the techniques described on page 13, pay particular attention to the signs listed on the next page. If you do spot any of these signs, try not to panic as most changes to a breast are normal or because of a benign breast condition rather than a sign of breast cancer. Just make sure that see your doctor as soon as you can.

Signs to look out for when checking your breasts:

- A lump or thickening in an area of the breast;
- A change in the size, shape or feel of a breast;
- Dimpling of the skin;
- A change in the shape of your nipple, particularly if it turns in, sinks into the breast, or has an irregular shape;
- A blood-stained discharge from the nipple;
- A rash on a nipple or surrounding area;
- A swelling or lump in your armpit;
- Sharp shooting pains in the breast; and
- Signs of fatigue.

Wednesday, 18th February 2015

Morning: Phlebotomy day! Going for my bloods always comes around so quickly but waiting for the results seems to take FOREVER! I'm hoping, because I've had the injections, that my bloods will be on their best behaviour. Because I'm experiencing so many different side effects and feeling like crap permanently, it's hard to tell whether how I'm feeling is because my bloods are low or I'm just experiencing the after effects of the last treatment.

Afternoon: After what seems like days, Sally rang. My stomach churned as I answered the phone to hear, "Sarah, I'm really sorry but your bloods are too high so you can't have chemo." My mind is in turmoil and I'm so frustrated. I'm trying my best not to cry. How can this be possible? How can they be too low one week and too high the next? Sally explained it's to do with the GCSF injections I have been having.

White blood cells are part of our immune system and fight infection. When the number of white cells in your blood is low, you are more likely to get infections because there are fewer white cells to fight off bacteria. It also makes some stem cells move from the bone marrow into the blood. Stem cells are the cells in the bone marrow from which red blood cells, white cells and platelets develop and this is why chemotherapy had to be postponed.

Whenever this happened, all my attempts at being positive and strong fell apart. I was trying so hard to be resilient but I was feeling brittle and helpless. Despite my best efforts, whenever I came off the phone from a conversation like this, I would end up crying as I told Dave the bad news. It takes so much effort to stay positive mentally and becomes more difficult when your body starts to give up physically. Feeling like shit every single day and struggling to do the simple daily chores because you're so fatigued and in so much discomfort really takes it out of you. To be told your treatment has been cancelled again, meaning this horrible nightmare would go on for longer, seems like the last straw.

This time, it resulted in me having to start the injections again on the Friday and from then on I would be monitored more closely, meaning having to visit phlebotomy on Mondays AND Wednesdays to enable them to keep an eye on my blood count and prevent it from becoming too high or low again.

This meant chemo now wouldn't be due to finish until April, all being well (originally it was due to finish mid-March). It doesn't sound like much but when you are counting the weeks, every small delay seems massive.

Monday came and my blood count was OK…so I could stop the injections. It felt like it took a lifetime to get to Wednesday, when I would have more tests to see if I could go ahead with the next treatment. I was so anxious and couldn't wait for the call from Sally, so I called her. My bloods had just come back and they had showed a little on the low side but nothing too serious to prevent me from having chemo. I was back on track!

This was my fourth dose of weekly chemo, meaning I'd only got five left if everything else went to plan. As I've said before, chemo was a bit easier when I was only having Paclitaxel. I still felt tired but didn't have the nausea. Having said that, over the few weeks since starting on the Carboplatin and Paclitaxel, I had noticed lots of changes in my body: puffy eyes, dehydrated skin, lines and wrinkles, age spots around my eyes, more intense hot and cold sweats, no taste buds, pale and grey skin, severe headaches, sore eyes which were sensitive to light — I found wearing an eye mask whenever I slept helped.

I had actually returned to work before my fourth treatment, so I slept as it was happening — chemo had actually become my day of rest! Because I had a bed at every chemo session from then on I found it quite relaxing once the IV was in!

It wasn't long before it was phlebotomy day again. My bloods had come back OK on Monday, showing no signs of concern. However, on the Wednesday it was a completely different story. My blood count was low so chemo would have to be cancelled

The Shock Factor

AGAIN! This was becoming a concern due to having to cancel the weekly treatments of Paclitaxel. It was important that I still had this drug, as its job was to stop cancer cells separating into two new cells, blocking the growth of the cancer. When I spoke with my oncologist on the phone she was unsure as it to whether or not they were going to give me the last dose of Carboplatin because of the impact it was having on my blood counts. Mentally I couldn't take any more disappointment. My body was running on reserves and I still had four treatments to go. To make the situation worse, I had picked up a cold and came down with the symptoms the following day (the planned chemo day). As the days went on my cold worsened, making the side effects feel 10 times worse. I spent the next few days in bed, resting to get myself better for the Thursday. It was so draining having to juggle dealing with side effects with the mental stress of not knowing from one week to the next whether chemo would go ahead.

It was that time of the week again and I had managed to get myself better. However, as before it was hard to tell whether or not I was still experiencing symptoms from the cold or whether they were actually side effects from the chemo treatment. Chemo was good to go ahead as my blood tests came back clear, which meant if they did decide to give me the Carboplatin, it would be my last one! It was amazing the negative impact treatment being postponed had on my morale, making me look forward to chemo… because, given a choice, I would much prefer to put up with the nasty side effects anyway, just to get it over and done with so I could feel and look human again!

Thursday, 12th March 2015

Chemo day – last day of Carboplatin!

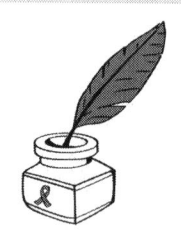

When we arrived at the hospital there was a bit of a delay to see my oncologist, meaning I couldn't wait any longer for my weekly treat. My chemo cap took me to my happy place…I would completely indulge in my warm drink, focusing on how delicious every little sip was, taking my mind off everything that was going on for that moment. Cap finished, I came back from my happy place to hear my name being called. We had a lengthy chat with Dr Horsley about my side effects and my treatment plan options. I described how I'd been feeling over the last couple of weeks, outlining my frustrations that my weekly chemo had been postponed twice. I also explained my concerns about the impact it would have on my body long-term. Dr Horsley wasn't sure whether we should carry on with the last Carboplatin and take the risk of treatment being postponed again. However, after coming this far and although I didn't know how well this extra treatment may work, I wanted to have the last dose to make sure I don't reproach myself later on, not knowing whether or not that last treatment may have prevented it recurring. I made the decision to have it, even though I was not looking forward to feeling like crap for the next seven days as well as having to have those awful steroids and injections. However, I always looked for a positive and, after the last Carboplatin, I would only need to have four more doses of the Paclitaxel — Yay!

> *Monday, 16th March 2016*
>
> *Woke up feeling really bad this morning – aching muscles from the injections I've been having to boost my white blood cells, fatigued from not sleeping for the last three nights, nausea and generally just feeling like crap. My make-up is taking me a lot longer to apply; even the simplest of things that I found effortless before, like applying mascara, makes my arm ache from holding it up, which means I now have to rest in-between applications. Brushing my teeth and cleansing my face is such a big effort. Showering – squeezing shower gel from the bottle, washing and drying my body – is so tiring. I now feel like a young person in an old person's body. My poor body is looking battered and bruised after being stabbed from all the needles – I'm feeling like a pin cushion and can't bear to hear the words 'Sharp scratch' anymore!*

Over the next two weeks my treatment went smoothly without any delays! As I was drawing closer to the end of treatment, I had noticed the hair on my eyebrows and eyelashes disappear; my precious hair was falling out strand by strand, leaving bald patches in my eyebrows and gaps in my eyelashes. It became a struggle to apply my mascara without painting my eyelid. I held out as long as I could but there was one only one thing for it…the false eyelashes and eyebrow pencil had to be called in!

The following day I stopped at Boots on my way to a meeting and bought some eyelashes. The plan was that I would have plenty of time to put them on to give me a bit of a boost. After being stuck in traffic I arrived fashionably late to the meeting venue and still without eyelashes on. There was no way I could turn up for the meeting without my eyelashes, so I parked in the furthest parking bay I could and prepared for 'Mission Eyelash'! It was very rare that I wore false eyelashes because my eyelashes were pretty long naturally and, once I applied my three layers of mascara, they looked even longer, resulting in everyone seeing my eyelashes before they actually saw me! Wearing false eyelashes irritated my eyes and always made them appear smaller. However, right now I was very thankful false eyelashes were in existence. Before pulling down the car visor I looked in every direction to make sure nobody was around. Coast clear, I removed the eyelashes from the packaging. Picking up the first eyelash very gently, making sure I didn't stretch it as it released from the self-adhesive, I sized up the eyelash by positioning it just above where my eyelashes used to be. As I placed it on the edge of the eyelid and removed the lid from the tube of glue I became aware that the glue had a very interesting fishy aroma! Pulling out the glue stick, I ran a thin layer on the root of the false eyelash, taking a deep breath before sticking it into position. Phew! It went on perfectly. I removed the second eyelash from the packaging, applied the glue, and started to place it in position. However, this is the eye that I struggle to close whilst keeping the other one open, making it a bit difficult to see where I was actually applying the eyelash. I took a deep breath and struggled to position it correctly. The more I focused on getting it right, the more my hand started to shake. All this time I was becoming more aware that I was now running even later for my meeting. However, I couldn't just turn up with one eyelash on! My body started to get hot and I had to take off my wig as I felt the beginnings of a hot flush (another generous free gift/side effect courtesy of the big C!) At this point, the car park had started to fill up and, even though there were lots of free spaces elsewhere, I became like a magnet, attracting cars to all the spaces around me. However, I had past caring what people thought and, by the time I actually got my last eyelash and put my wig back on, they wouldn't recognise me anyway! After three attempts I finally got my second eyelash on — not positioned quite as perfectly as the first, however, to the untrained eye you would never have known. I just had to hope it stayed in position for my meeting. Wig back on and 'Operation Eyelash' complete, I headed off to my meeting ready to conquer the world!

Despite it not being the most pleasant experience, I had never had a problem with the nurses finding a vein. However, this all changed in my last but one chemo session. They struggled to get the cannula in, realising one of my worst nightmares of having to be cannulated more than once. Up until that point my veins had played ball but, to be fair, if I was a vein I would have run away a long time ago, being pricked by a sharp scratch every week! It took five attempts before she finally found a vein and, even then, it was the tiniest vein. Normally they would put in a picc line if this happened (a picc line is a long, thin, flexible tube which is inserted into a vein and can stay in place between treatments). However, because I only had one more chemo after this one it wouldn't be worth it.

Over the next few days I started to think more about my last chemo and how good I was going to be feeling not having all those nasty chemicals in my body. Each time I imagined feeling normal I got rushes of excitement. As the evening before my last chemo drew closer I was very excited. It didn't feel real. I was feeling much stronger than I had been and was ready to take on my final chemo. I just hoped my veins would man up and didn't disappear again!

Alongside the harsh impact that the weeks of chemo treatment had on my body, I also had the fear of undergoing a double mastectomy at the back of my mind. I decided to meet this challenge head-on by arranging a 'Boobs Voyage' party. Initially, this was supposed to take place a few weeks after chemo treatment finished but, because treatment had been postponed a few times, it was now going to take place the evening of my last chemo. Not the best planning but there was no way I was going to back out of THIS party!

Thursday, 2nd April 2015

It's Chemo Thursday! Not any old Chemo Thursday – my last one!! And it's my Boob Voyage party – whoop whoop! Just been shopping to get all the balloons, party accessories and some flowers and Easter cakes for the nurses. My lovely friend, Nikki, lush husband and gorgeous daughter have showered me with beautiful flowers this morning. Dave's also bought me a bottle of Veuve to have as a special drink tonight. If I'm going to mix chemo with champagne, it's got to be the good stuff! Feel like I'm walking on cloud 9. I keep having rushes of excitement every time I realise it's actually my last EVER chemo.

Unfortunately, things were not going to plan on the last chemo day. The chemo unit were running late so my chemo was delayed until 3pm. I couldn't believe it. I mean, didn't they know I had a Boob Voyage party to go to! I'm probably the only

The Shock Factor 57

patient that's ever had a party a few hours after chemo! When they finally called to tell me they were ready, I ran as quickly as I could in my pink Dr Martens back to the hospital! I thought it would help get the veins pumping. It helped, but I still had to be cannulated twice — at least it wasn't five times! Because of the delays, I wasn't going to be leaving until gone six. The panic set in as all I could think about was that we still hadn't decorated the cabin where my party was to be held and everything I had bought was in the house. Once again, my best friend, Nikki, came to the rescue and sorted it all out. As always, she was there in my hour of need. I can't tell you how much it helped to have a good friend by my side throughout this whole nightmare. She was always on hand to help in any way, from picking Lillie up and looking after her, popping in to see how I was, helping me choose my wig (and give it a blow dry!) and even leaving little presents on the doorstep to cheer me up. Because of Nikki we got to celebrate 'Boobs Voyage' in style — but more about that in Chapter Seven.

All through my treatment, I had been imagining how it would feel once my last chemo was over. In my head I expected to magically return to how I had felt before it all started. It was not like that…not like that at all.

Three days after my last chemo, it was Easter Sunday and I was so tired and nauseous, with frequent headaches (I was getting up in the night to take codeine phosphate because of the pain) and still no taste buds — a bit different to the previous year when I was up early with Lillie and full of energy! I expected to be feeling so happy and excited, however, it was the complete opposite: mentally and physically fatigued, feeling and looking like crap and fed up. It didn't feel fair after having just got through the most horrendous few months.

TOP TIPS TO HELP WHEN YOU HAVE NO TASTE BUDS
- Drink plenty of water;
- Rinse or brush teeth before eating;
- Try stronger tasting foods;
- Season your food with different flavours; and
- Eat warm foods as they have more taste than cold food.

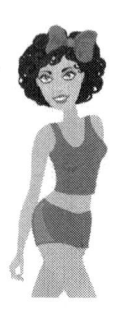

The treatment had really taken it out of me with countless restless nights' sleep, blocked sinuses and a lot of blood up my nose — this usually happened for a few days after chemo. Normally, I didn't feel as bad after the smaller dose of drugs but this time, after my last chemo, I felt as though I had been hit by a truck, as though I had had an intensive dose. My body was feeling the full impact and I noticed that I was breathless by the time I got to the top of the stairs, something that was never the case previously. Also, my periods had stopped in the last two months, so my hormones had been all over the place and my body had started to go into early menopause. This resulted in the delightful side effect of hot flushes, which drove me crazy. My skin seemed to age even more and became so dry; my eyes were puffy and very sensitive to light.

I felt so much older than my age and couldn't wait to feel like a 33-year-old again! There and then I vowed never to complain about my periods ever again when my body resumed back to normality, whenever that was going to be.

My thoughts kept returning to the possibility of me dying and asking myself 'What if it's spread?' I'd been experiencing new and different pains and twinges, feeling more tired than normal and coughing a lot. It's always in the back of your mind, regardless of how much you try to be positive. The trick for me was to try to ignore it but there were times when it wandered into my conscious mind and I had no control of it. I had so much to live for. I would beat this.

It wasn't long before there were signs of hope and my body showed small steps of recovery. I started to wake up a bit more refreshed, my skin was looking fresher, I wasn't looking as tired and the puffiness around my eyes has gone down, ever so slightly but it was noticeable to me, so I could actually see my eyes! I even noticed my toenails starting to look white and healthy again. In particular, I was really excited about my hair growing back. Starting to see my body slowly changing and having little glimpses of what it was going to feel like to feel normal again filled me with elation.

Despite the amazing support of my friends and family, I felt scared and alone after months of treatment. Suddenly it felt as though I was expected to live a normal life again — however I wasn't sure how? For the last 12 months I'd had to adapt my lifestyle to accommodate my diagnosis and treatment and learn how to live with breast cancer. Now I had to teach myself how to deal with life after breast cancer and what was now a 'new normal'.

Thursday, 9th April 2015

Stayed at my mum and dad's overnight. It felt very strange waking up knowing it was Thursday but no chemo! My mum suggested we go to Southport beach. It was a beautiful morning and I thought it would be a perfect way to spend my first Thursday after finishing chemo. We had a lovely day but I started to get a bit emotional after reading some of the lovely comments people had written on my Facebook post about going to the beach. While I stood in the queue waiting to get some chips, I felt isolated as I looked on from the outside, taking everything in. I didn't belong in this world that I was once a part of, the world I felt comfortable to be in just before my diagnosis. Last week I was having chemotherapy and, one week later, I'm standing in a queue waiting for some chips. A wave of overwhelm and emotions flooded over me as I realised I missed my chemo partner – a part of me was missing and I should be spending the time with Dave and Lillie as a family. I sent a text to Dave to let him know I was missing him and that not having him with me felt like a part of me was missing. He replied saying he felt exactly the same. Of course, my mum, Lillie and I had a great time and I thoroughly enjoyed spending our time together eating chips and ice-cream. Most of all, it was wonderful seeing Lillie so happy. There has been a big change in her ever since we told her Mummy no longer has to have special medicine. I think it affected her more than I realised. For the last few months Dave has done a fantastic job of taking on the mummy and daddy role but I think she's very happy to have both mummy and daddy back! When we arrived home I was elated to see Dave. He gave me the biggest cuddle and, as I was clutched in his arms, my eyes began to well. Before I knew it, tears were streaming down my face. The realisation of what I had just been through the last few months has just hit me.

CHAPTER SIX

Hair Today…Gone Tomorrow

Your hair is something that helps define who you are, makes a statement and, especially for women, is a crucial part of your look. The risk of losing your hair is a big fear for most women who are diagnosed with cancer. I was no different. Ever since I could remember I had been so proud of my dark hair, which I always wore long. Who would I be without it? Because of hair loss being such a significant issue, I have decided to dedicate a whole chapter to the subject.

After my diagnosis I immediately decided to take control of the cancer before it took control of me and one of the ways I would do this would be by having my beautiful long hair cut into three different styles over time, each one shorter then the last, before it started to fall out. My thinking behind this was so that the hair loss process would be less of a shock and hopefully it would lessen the trauma.

I had been diagnosed on a Tuesday and by the Thursday of that same week my long locks had been cut and styled into a neat bob! Although it was very distressing to have my ponytail cut off I really liked my new style. It helped me to accept my diagnosis, and made me feel stronger and ready to take on the awful disease I was about to face.

It was most likely that my hair would fall out three weeks after chemo started so I didn't have long to experiment before I lost it — I didn't waste any time! After the bob, the second style I had was a graduated bob; there wasn't much difference between the two only that the graduated bob was a lot shorter at the back and longer at the jawline. It was the final style, a pixie cut, I found the most difficult as this was the shortest my hair had ever been and it didn't feel like me. However, I did get a lot of complimentary comments! Despite the positive remarks from everyone, it took me right up until my hair started to fall out to get used to the style and then, when I finally lost my hair, I regretted not embracing it, making the most of it and enjoying the hair I had left.

TOP TIPS FOR PREPARING FOR AND DEALING WITH HAIR LOSS:

- Use a soft brush to comb hair;
- Cut hair short before chemotherapy to prevent the weight of long hair pulling on the scalp; and
- Wear a hairnet at night to help collect loose hair and prevent your hair from becoming tangled.

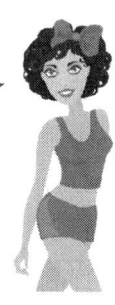

Wig Shopping

Two weeks before I had my first chemotherapy treatment, I had decided to go wig shopping to make sure I was prepared for when I started to lose my hair. As I said, I had been told it would be two to three weeks after starting treatment that my hair was likely to start falling out.

Where to find a good wig:

- Your local NHS wig supplier;
- A wig supplier or salon;
- Hairdressers who supply wigs; and
- Internet or postal shopping.

My friends, Lillie and I had decided the time had come to go wig shopping; we had planned to go to a particular wig shop in Manchester that had been recommended to one of my friends. However we later found out it didn't open on Saturdays and it was the only one we had researched (Top tip — choose at least three to begin with just in case!) We then had a look on Google at other places but there were very few that were open on a Saturday. We eventually found one that looked OK and gave them a call to see whether an appointment was necessary; it was, but luckily the lady had just had a cancellation. My friend had offered to chauffeur me there so I felt like a celebrity! It was a hairdresser that specialised in wig fitting, however you would not really know this as it just looked like a normal hair salon.

When we got there the lady was running a bit late, so we found a gorgeous cake shop next door and decided to have afternoon tea with a glass of prosecco to make our wig shopping day a memorable occasion. We headed back to the salon after consuming a ridiculous amount of cakes and sandwiches. I was ready for the wig parade to begin!

I had gone there not really knowing what style I wanted but had done some research into the variety of wigs that were on the market and how they are sized.

Wigs come in three basic sizes: large, average and petite — most women (90-95%) will wear an average size cap.

How to measure for a wig

Temple to Temple — Start at your temple (which is on the side of your head, behind your eye but before your hairline), and bring the tape measure around the back of your head to reach the other temple.

Ear to Ear — Lay the end of the tape about a half inch above your little crease (where glasses rest) at the top of your ear, between the ear and the head. Bring the tape across the top of your head to meet the other ear, without touching the ear, at the same point.

Forehead to Nape — Start the tape from the centre of the front of your hairline, to the hairline at the nape of the neck. If you have little or no hair, lay your index, third, and ring finger flat against your forehead just about at the brow bone. At the top of the three fingers would be a good straight point. Measure until about an inch below the small bone at the bottom of the skull

Wig measurements

Cap Size	Temple to Temple	Ear to ear	Front to Nape
petite	21"	13"	13¾"
average	21½"	13½"	14¼"
large	23"	14"	15¼"

Basically there are three main materials used in wigs: synthetic, heat-friendly synthetic and human hair.

Synthetic high quality wigs look natural and have the benefit of retaining their shape, meaning there is very little styling. However, the negative is that you cannot put heated devices such as a hair dryer, straighteners or any other styling equipment on the synthetic fibres. Care also has to be taken when cooking, especially when putting food in and taking it out of the oven! My mum had a synthetic wig which had a fringe, however, during a few weeks of wearing it whilst cooking, it got shorter and shorter because she had singed it that many times. She only ever remembered about it when she heard the sound of her hair starting to shrivel and smelt a distinct, sharp odour of burnt hair around the kitchen. Synthetic wigs generally tend to last 4–6 months (worn everyday) if looked after properly.

Heat-friendly synthetic wigs can be styled using heat (maximum of 350 degrees). This will allow you to style your 'hair' from straight to curly. The negative is that they are not as easy to style as a human hair wig and don't retain their shape as well. However, they are a good alternative if you want something that is affordable and that you can style!

Human Hair wigs give you the same versatility as real hair, allowing you to wash it and style it exactly how you want. However the negative is that it requires a lot more styling and maintenance because it is made with real hair. They can sometimes become dry and brittle if not maintained properly and are very expensive.

I had my heart set on a human hair wig. However, the wig allowance you get from the NHS was NEVER going to cover even a quarter of the cost. After trying on numerous wigs in a variety of styles (good and bad) I was running out of options. The wig I really liked was a beautiful long brown human hair wig which was just under £500! (I only had £95 from the NHS.) I didn't feel I could justify this amount of money on a wig (even though I had cancer), especially as I would only be wearing it for about 11 months.

The disappointment set in as I started to give up hope and accept the dream of getting a human hair wig was not going to be a reality. I had tried on a couple of really lovely synthetic wigs but the downside was that they weren't heat friendly which meant I didn't have the option to style it — a 'deal-breaker' for me. Just when I thought I had explored all my options, the lady in the salon told me about a second-hand human hair wig that had been used as a demonstration wig at a few hairdressing shows. I kept an open and positive mind. (I had absolutely no idea where the lady was getting the wigs from; she just kept disappearing into a small cupboard in the corner of the salon and then appearing with different wigs — it was like Aladdin's cave!) She pulled out this GINGER wig (definitely not a colour I would normally go for). However, I was still hopeful. As she placed it on my head, the first thing that came to mind was Worzel Gummidge! Not only was it ginger, it was different lengths! My open mind and positivity started to fade very fast… this was not what I had imagined.

Luckily I had Lindsey and Nicola with me, who are both hairdressers. They said it was fixable and could be transformed into something beautiful (they obviously saw something I definitely didn't). The only positive I could see at this point was that it was only going to cost £100, which meant I would only have to put £5 towards it! It was not as long I would have liked or the right colour, but my friend said she could fix it. The ginger wig it was then!

All I could do was giggle about the whole experience and the fact I had come away with a wig that looked nothing like I had imagined! However, it is something I will always remember and a very funny story to tell and share with you.

When we got home, we went to my friend's salon to have a proper look at my new wig. When we did a full examination, it had big chunks cut out from the underneath (it looked like a child had been using it as a 'Girl's World'). This meant it would have to be cut shorter to make it even. The more I was wearing the wig, the more I got used to the colour and eventually made the big decision to embrace being ginger for a couple of weeks.

By the time I got home I was drained and my head was so sore and tender from trying on so many wigs! I never knew wig shopping would be so exhausting!

TOP WIG SHOPPING TIPS

- Go shopping 2–3 weeks before you start treatment;
- If possible choose a minimum of three wigs shops in the same area to give you more variety;
- Make your wig shopping experience fun and memorable - go with family and friends, go shopping, drink prosecco, have lunch or afternoon tea;
- Experiment with different styles and colours - now is your time to try something completely new;
- Choose the right colour for your skin tone (low lights and high lights give a good variation of colour); and
- Get an adjustable size.

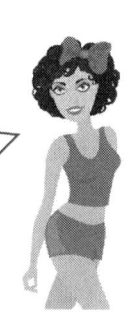

Losing my hair

It was a normal Monday morning as I was sat with my little girl having breakfast and reading together. That cold, dull wintery day when I felt an itch and reached up to scratch my head to find hair in my fingers will forever be etched in my memory. Even though I knew it was going to happen and had mentally prepared myself and taken control by having my hair cut from very long to, eventually, a pixie cut, it was still a massive shock to see it falling out through my fingers. This was a milestone in my journey, a milestone in my battle with cancer, to know that in a few days my hair, the hair that had been part of my life and my identity from the day I was born, would be gone and soon I would be looking like a boiled egg!

That morning I even had to ask my best friend to take Lillie to school because I just didn't feel I could speak to any of the mums at the school gates. It was the first time since being diagnosed that I felt sorry for myself, so much so that I didn't want to get dressed or put my make-up on. I just didn't feel like being in anyone else's company apart from my own.

That day I had a Christmas lunch booked with a group of ladies (from 'Sue France, Creative Connecting in Cheshire' networking group) at Gusto in Knutsford.

I was unsure whether I wanted to attend; I wasn't feeling very glamorous, had been looking tired for a few days since chemo due to sleep deprivation from the steroids, and had now started to lose my hair so didn't feel I could be bothered to put my war paint on to make myself look like me.

An hour later I needed to give my editor, Sian-Elin, a call to confirm a meeting and when we got talking I explained that my hair had started falling out and that I wasn't going to attend the lunch because of the way I was feeling. She said I should go as it would do me the world of good — so I did! After I got off the call to Sian-Elin I felt so much better, so I took myself upstairs, pulled out one of my favourite dresses, spent extra time doing my make-up and then I did what is called an affirmation; I told myself that I was a confident, strong, beautiful woman and I felt fabulous. Anybody who has tried saying affirmations will know you feel really silly and very uncomfortable the first time you attempt it. However, it makes you feel fantastic and becomes more normal the more you do and say it. Affirmation done, I set off for Gusto.

When I arrived, a few familiar faces greeted me, Sian-Elin being one of them. Unfortunately she had the starting of a cold so we were not able to come into contact with each other. The most natural thing for me was to greet her with a hug, especially after what had happened that morning and our chat earlier. This was another moment of reality — recognising your immune system is so fragile that you have to protect yourself and this sometimes means not being able to have close physical contact with the people you love and care about, occasionally when you most need it.

I was very happy that I made the decision to go to the event as it was so lovely to see everyone and make some new friends. It was just what was I needed to boost my confidence again and get me back to being that strong, independent women and feeling that I could do this.

As the days went on I started to lose more hair; each morning when I woke up it would look like a furry animal had been sleeping on my pillow and I would find hair constantly all over the house as well as in my food and cups of coffee — even poor Lillie used to complain! As well as being extremely distressing, losing my hair become an annoyance, especially at meal times; I didn't realise it but my hair was falling out while I was preparing the food so that when we sat down to eat, poor Dave and Lillie would be finding strands in their food. Although it was clean, there is nothing worse than finding another person's hair in your food!

I found myself, whenever I was at home or in the bathroom, pulling out all the loose hairs. It was so therapeutic and helped ease the tension and pain in my head from the pressure on the hair follicle.

Enough is enough! It was now Friday and I had made the decision to have all my hair shaved off as seeing bald patches on my head was making me feel worse. As soon as I got up on Saturday morning I was ready to go for it. Of course, I was feeling very nervous and apprehensive. Few of us know what we will look like bald and it wasn't long before I was going to find out!

Saturday, 14th November, 2014

Dave had everything prepared in the bathroom and luckily we had a professional pair of hair clippers that Dave uses for his own hair. I took a seat and prepared myself for what was about to come. Tomorrow I will be wearing my ginger wig for the first time. I took a deep breath as Dave turned on the clippers; as he came closer they get louder and louder. He started at the base of my neck and slowly moved them up my head. My hair follicles were so sore and sensitive it was as though I could feel the clippers pulling out each and every strand of hair. The tears rolled down my face as my hair fell in small mounds all around me. My beautiful hair, my identity, taken away from me just like that.

Throughout the process, Dave tried his best to comfort me, cracking a couple of jokes to make me feel better. Before I knew it, he was on to the last bit of hair. I took one final deep breath as I watched the very last lock of hair fall to the floor. My hair that has been such a big part of my life and such an important part of my identity was gone so quickly, lifeless in a big pile on the floor.

I couldn't help but think back to that moment, 12 years earlier, when I shaved my mum's hair as she was going through breast cancer. Poor Lillie was there when I was having mine shaved, but didn't really take much notice until I was bald. She looked at me as if I was an alien, wondering what on earth Daddy had done to Mummy!

After I got over the initial shock of seeing my hair all over the floor, I felt so relieved and happy that I had made the decision to have my head shaved. Having bald patches and waking up every morning with hair on my pillow was so soul-destroying that it made me feel fragile and more ill. Being bald actually made me feel strong again and back in control. I decided I now had to accept my hair had gone and embrace my new look! At first I couldn't stop feeling my smooth scalp and looking at myself in the mirror (GI Jane came to mind).

The next few days after shaving my hair, my scalp became sore and I had a cluster of red, raised blisters on the top of my head. Over the next few days I treated them with 100% inner leaf Aloe Vera gelly, applying it 3–4 times a day. This reduced the redness, helping to take out the sting and ease the pain. After three days they started to heal.

Whenever I was at home I wore a beanie hat to keep my head warm and to make me feel more comfortable. Although Dave was very accepting of me having no hair and loved me no matter what I looked like, it was something I needed to do to make me feel better. It was the height of winter when my hair fell out so my head got very cold, especially at night time, and my blue beanie hat was my constant accessory — it wasn't long before we created a bond that could never be broken and my treasured blue beanie became my comfort blanket!

As the days went on I got used to having no hair. Showering was much easier and quicker as I didn't need to spend time washing and conditioning my hair — however it did take a few showers with my head being covered in a lather of soap suds before I realised that I didn't need as much shampoo as I only had my scalp to wash! Getting ready was quicker as I didn't have to style my hair, only my wig. Actually I really enjoyed styling my wig. My friend who is a Hairdressing lecturer kindly let me borrow a mannequin head to hold my wig and keep it looking good. (It was quite funny because my 'new friend' the mannequin also had a bald head so we looked like twin sisters!) I didn't really do much with my wig at first but, as the time went on, I loved experimenting by putting Velcro rollers in and curling it with the tongs. I also enjoyed blow-drying it as I could actually style it properly — with my own hair I struggled to dry it evenly at the back, so I would have beautifully blow-dried hair at the sides but God only knows what it looked like from behind.

I was so happy that I had managed to get a human hair wig (even if it was ginger and had been sat in a box for an eternity!) It had taken me three weeks to get used to the feeling of wearing a wig and, although it had a soft netting inside, fitted securely and felt comfortable. However, it often made my scalp itch and I couldn't help but want to rip it off at times, especially if I was somewhere where it was really warm. The problem was I didn't think it would have done my street cred any good if I had ripped it off in the middle of the supermarket, or a restaurant whilst having dinner, although there were many times I felt like it, especially when I was experiencing hot flushes from chemotherapy treatment.

After embracing being strawberry blonde (ginger) for a couple of weeks, I decided it was time for a change and chose to go a vibrant red. (This was another benefit to a human hair wig — you can change the colour!) My friend had never had any experience in dying or styling wigs before so this was as completely new to her as it was to me. The biggest concern was how she was going to colour the hair without dying the scalp bright red! I have to say it was the most bizarre experience, holding the mannequin's neck to keep it still whilst my friend attempted to apply the colour. We sat 'her' to one side while the colour took in the hope that the colour could be removed easily from the netting (fake scalp) without it staining. All we could both do was laugh about the whole situation — laughing is the best medicine ever! As my friend held my wig over the kitchen sink I started to feel apprehensive. We both took a deep breath as the dye washed away and kept everything crossed that it hasn't dyed the scalp. Phew, we could finally breathe as the netting gradually returned to its original colour. We were both giddy and excited about the next stage… restyle!

At that stage the wig was shoulder length. I had decided I wanted it cut into a bob. For the cutting part I put the wig on, as it would be much easier to cut. I have to say, putting a wig that's cold and wet onto a beautifully warm scalp is a breath-taking experience! After my wig had been cut and blow-dried it was time for the big reveal. Wow, I was completely blown away! The wig felt brand new and was a total transformation. It looked and felt gorgeous. Yet again, I was so glad I made the decision to have a human hair wig; it felt just like my own hair. In one evening I had gone from looking like Worzel Gummidge to resembling someone from a Vidal Sassoon advert. I couldn't thank my friend enough as she had well and truly excelled in her duty!

The next morning I got up full of excitement about having a girly day out with my friend. I put my make-up on, including some red lips (red lipstick made me feel like superwoman and ready for anything), my favourite leopard-print dress (leopard always made me feel sexy, hair or no hair!) and, last but not least, my wig! I loved the fact my wig was styled and ready to go — I felt fabulous! I practically skipped to the school gates that morning with Lillie. Hair loss and wearing a wig wasn't all that bad after all!

At some point I knew my hair was going to grow back (well, I was 99.9% sure) and in much better condition than before. That didn't mean I couldn't have some fun in the meantime. Over the months, I embraced my wig and became spontaneous with my colour choices by having a few different shades of red. I had never been able to experiment like this with my own hair due the risk of damage it would cause long-term. However, I had nothing to lose with my wig.

There was some interesting hair colouring experiences, my last one being the funniest. I had to go into the college were my friend worked because she couldn't come to the house. When I got there she was running a little late and, because of the colour I had wanted, the wig required bleaching first. For anyone reading this who has had his or her hair bleached, you will know it's a long process, so as you can imagine it took much longer than we thought. This meant I was going to be in the salon a lot longer than I had accounted for. Due to having a training session planned with one of my team members, I had to leave before we had finished. Long story short, my friend had to apply the final colour after the bleaching process and I had to go home with my wig in a plastic bag! It was the most bizarre hair colouring experience I had ever had. When I got home, I got so caught up in my training that I completely lost track of time, forgetting that my wig was still in my handbag. When I finally remembered, the colour should have been washed off two hours previously. I have never run up the stairs so fast in my life! I was so scared as I carefully took it out of the plastic bag, in case the hair just fell out everywhere. It was my only wig! What would I do? (Well, I did have this beautiful turban I bought at the same time as I got my wig, which I had as a backup in a worst-case scenario.) Luckily it was all fine; the colour was beautiful and (shall we say) 'vibrant', not surprising given the time it had been on for!

As well as my lack of hair and my wig creating lots of funny and memorable moments for me, it did for Lillie too…one of which was Mummy pretending to be Gollum from the 'Lord of the Rings'. Just in case you have no idea who he is, he is a small, slimy creature, emaciated, gaunt and pale with a few strands of hair. Also at the time I lost my hair, the world had gone 'Frozen' mad — so much so, I knew the 'Let it go' lyrics off by heart because we always had it on in the car. One day, Lillie wanted to listen to it while she was in the bath, so I decided I would create my own version along the lines of "I don't care if I've got no hair." At that point I pulled off my wig and finished off with "being bald never bothered me anyway!" Lillie giggled so much that this became a firm favourite entertainment at bath time!

Each day I looked for the silliest ways I could entertain my precious little girl just to hear her laugh and to see her beautiful smile in the hope I was turning what could have so easily been memories of sadness into memories of happiness.

There have also been many funny wig moments when I have entertained other people without realising. One time I thought my wig was on properly only to find out, when I caught a glimpse of myself in the mirror, it was sitting quite far back, making my forehead seem extra-large! Another time, a month after finishing treatment, I attended Lillie's sports day and entered the mums' 100m running race, completely forgetting I was wearing a wig and nearly lost it at the finish line! I also nearly lost my wig a couple of times when the wind really picked up. I walked around with my hand on my head, holding on to my wig for dear life, at the same time trying not to draw attention to myself!

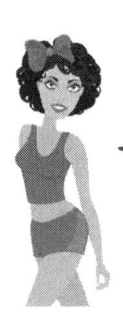

> **TOP TIPS TO AVOID WIG DISASTERS:**
> - When it is windy wear a hat or scarf;
> - Always carry a mirror in your handbag to check your wig is positioned correctly; and
> - Use double-sided tape or clips to keep it in place.

Wearing a wig has been an interesting experience, allowing me to experiment with different styles and colours, which I would never have had the courage to do with my own hair. The experience also provided lots of memorable and embarrassing moments. However, I am glad it was only a temporary measure and am so happy to now have my own hair back — you don't really appreciate it until you lose it.

Your hair usually starts to grow back after a few months of finishing treatment and, after 3–6 months, you are likely to have a full head of hair (however, it very much depends on the individual).

I have been very lucky with my hair and how quickly it has grown. It started to grow back a few days after my double mastectomy operation. I remember getting my friend, Lyndsey, to bring her clippers into the hospital to shave off all the new wispy bits of hair. (I wouldn't advise you do this unless you have your own private room and don't tell the nursing staff…. sshhhh!) I do believe that by shaving regularly it has encouraged my hair to grow much faster.

Be prepared for your hair to come back a different colour or texture. I had a few grey hairs before losing my hair, but when it grew back they were a lot more noticeable. Nevertheless, the texture is lovely — very soft (like baby hair) and curly (I think I definitely got the Christie Perm — what the chemotherapy nurses at The Christie call it when your hair grows back curly after treatment!), extremely thick and healthier than before. I'm very excited to see how my hair continues to grow and what style it will grow into next.

Of course, it is not only the hair on your head that goes when you have chemotherapy. As I mentioned in the last chapter, you lose hair from places where you didn't even notice it existed (nose hair), places where, previously, you had found it a nuisance (armpits, arms, legs and bikini line), as well as your eyelashes and eyebrows.

> **TOP TIP**
> Take pictures of your hair at different stages when it's growing back and write down how many weeks between each photograph. It really helps when you think your hair hasn't grown much then you look at the last picture taken and realise its grown more than you think!

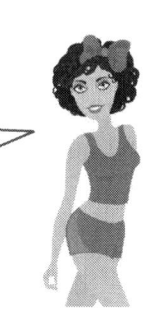

Now, I've said it before and I'll say it again, not everything about cancer is bad! Not having to shave, pluck and wax on a regular basis was fantastic! I found being completely hairless one of the highlights to my cancer journey. Due to having dark hair, hair removal was always on the maintenance list as a 'top priority'. However, whilst going through treatment it was one thing I didn't have to think about. I secretly wished that I would never see my body hair from my chin to my toes ever again; unfortunately my wish didn't come true, my hair grew back with a vengeance, with me getting a lot more than I had bargained for. This resulted in one hand being hairier than the other and me having a furry face! Luckily the hairs shed after a few weeks and my body's 'hairy-ness' returned back to how it was before chemo.

There are many things I don't miss about chemotherapy, but not having to shave, wax and pluck is one thing I do miss. Hair maintenance has resumed 'priority position' on a much more frequent level; my hair has grown back thicker and healthier than before, including my eyebrows and eyelashes and, although I would prefer not to have to use hair removal methods, I feel very grateful to have hair again.

CHAPTER SEVEN

All Things Boobs

I have always liked my boobs — no, loved my boobs — so the shock of getting breast cancer and knowing that I would have to have an operation and maybe have them removed had a huge impact on me. Because of this and the fact that, at the end of the day, this book is about my breast cancer journey, I have decided to dedicate a chapter to all things boobs.

Monday, 9th February 2015 – Pre-boobopic Day

It's the evening before I have my meeting with my surgeon to discuss my 'NEW' boobs! I'm very excited but also a bit unsure because I have no idea what to expect. I sort of imagine it might be like looking through a catalogue full of boobs, all different shapes and sizes, and I just choose the ones I want... or maybe not! I have no idea what size to go for, all I know is that I would like them to be not

> too big or too small and to sit comfortably and not be jigging around when I'm running. My appointment tomorrow feels very different to any previous hospital appointments because I know that what I'm going to discuss is positive and exciting but it also signifies my breast cancer journey coming to an end. By the time I have surgery I will have finished chemo...Woohoo! I have no idea how the surgery will be done but I feel very confident and relaxed that I'm in safe hands with Mr. Mahadev. I've heard great feedback from women who have had surgery done by him, about what a fantastic surgeon he is.

We arrived at the hospital, returning to the waiting room where we had sat just before I received my diagnosis (it was like returning to the scene of the crime). It gave me chills down my spine. I was much more relaxed this time and Dave and I were laughing and joking, discussing what boob size I should have. There was a moment when I felt a wave of sickness, but it only lasted for a few minutes; I think it was the fear of receiving bad news. I quickly reached in my bag for my red lipstick and compact mirror — it was definitely a red lipstick day! (I had found wearing red lipstick whenever I have been feeling vulnerable through my breast cancer journey has helped me to feel less vulnerable and more in control.) Lipstick on, I was ready — bring it on!

The first thing discussed was the operation procedure. Thankfully, Dave had put me on his company's private health insurance in January 2014, a few months before I got my diagnosis. This allowed me to be able to make the decision to go privately for my double mastectomy, which meant the insertions would only be made at the side of each breast instead of being cut in three different places and I would not have to have muscle taken from my back or thigh. I had been on the NHS for all my other treatments, including IVF and chemo, and have to say the treatment available and what I received from Leighton and The Christie hospital was incredible.

My operation was booked to take place on Monday 11th May 2015 if my chemotherapy went to plan without any more delays. As we talked through my hopes and expectations, I described to the surgeon about how I had envisaged the process involving me looking through a catalogue of boobs in different shapes and sizes before I made my choice. He laughed…a lot! I got the feeling nobody had gone in with this perception before!

It was explained to me that I would have to walk around with a drainage bag on one side of each breast for at least 10 days after my operation. Before discussing the size of my new boobs he needed to examine the breast with the tumours. It felt very uncomfortable having my husband, a Macmillan nurse and a surgeon all together in the same room whilst I was exposing myself. At this point I could only hope the conversation would keep flowing and not run dry, ending up in complete silence as I was getting undressed and as Mr Mahadev began to examine my breasts — that would be awkward!

Examination done… phew! Fully dressed, I made the decision to opt for a 32DD, playing it safe to prevent any long-term physical health issues such as back problems, due to my frame only being small. The thing I was most excited about was my boobs not moving when I would go running, as well as not having to wear a bra if I didn't want to. Since breastfeeding, my boobs had changed in shape and size; my surgeon confirmed this when he told me they were drooping a little bit and asked would I like a 'nipple lift' at the same time as my double mastectomy. At first I didn't know what to say and was taken aback by his question, however I respected his honesty and quickly answered with a YES — there had to be some benefits to having cancer!

Some questions you may want to ask your surgeon:

- Can I have an immediate breast reconstruction?
- Which reconstruction is best for me and why?
- What are the benefits, limitations and risks of this type of surgery?
- When can I have my surgery done?
- How long will I have to stay in hospital?
- What is the recovery time for this operation?
- How much pain is there likely to be?
- Can I keep my nipples?
- Can you show me where the scars will be and how big/long?
- Will I have scars elsewhere on my body?
- When can I exercise again?
- When will I be able to move about, walk and drive?
- Will reconstructive surgery delay my other cancer treatments, like chemotherapy and radiotherapy?
- Can you show me any photographs or images of your previous breast reconstructions?
- Can I speak to someone who has had the same type of reconstruction? (I met a girl the same age as me and found it very helpful chatting with her.)
- Do I need to wear any special bra after the operation?

Tuesday, 27th January 2015 – Sakana, Manchester

Today I attended a ladies' business lunch at Sakana. I met Rachel Halliwell, a well-known journalist. Rachel was doing a 30-minute presentation about her business and how it evolved, as well as showing us some of the great articles she had written. She was really interesting and I enjoyed listening to where she gets her inspiration from, especially as I'm writing my book and find it very difficult some days to put pen to paper and spend more time thinking about what to write as opposed to writing! After the presentation, my editor introduced me to Rachel. We got chatting and Rachel started to ask me about my breast cancer journey. She asked me how I felt, knowing I was going to lose my breasts through a mastectomy. It is a question I have not been asked before so I haven't really thought too much about it. I told her that when I first got diagnosed there were a few times I would catch myself in the mirror as I was getting out of the shower or whilst getting dressed, when I would look at my breasts and feel connected with them emotionally and would then feel grief that I was going to be losing them. I have always been very happy with the shape and size of my breasts and would never have wanted to change them given the choice. The big thing that fills me with sadness was that I knew I would no longer have the option to breastfeed in the future; I enjoyed breastfeeding so much (after I mastered the technique on how to do it and the sores on my nipples had healed). The intimate connection and bond you have with your baby, feeling them so close, is the most wonderful feeling in the world. Knowing I will no longer have that option has made me realise just how precious my boobs are and just how much my body is going to be put through. As time has gone on I have found myself starting to emotionally disconnect from my breasts and accept that they are now a detriment to my health and could cost me my life. I am now focusing on the excitement of having new boobs (ones which I can design myself). Losing my boobs is out of my control so I want to make the best out of my situation, take control and not let the cancer win. Having a 'Boob Voyage' pre-mastectomy party to celebrate the life, memories and journey that my boobs and me have been on will be my way of saying a sad farewell.

Fast forward and thankfully chemo had gone as planned, which meant my operation would go ahead on the original date. However, my 'Boob Voyage' party was now going to fall on the eve of my last day of chemo. The date for my 'Boob Voyage' had always been planned for Thursday, 2nd April, which was actually the day before Good Friday. Due to my chemotherapy treatment being postponed a couple of times because of my low blood count, it now meant that my party fell on the last day of chemo. I did wonder whether it was a good idea but I had already put the necessary arrangements into place and didn't want to cancel.

As I described in Chapter Five, on my last day of chemo, of all days, my treatment was delayed by two hours, which meant I wouldn't be treated until three o'clock. I couldn't believe it! I started to panic whilst working out the timings; it meant I wouldn't be arriving home until after seven and I still had to decorate the cabin ready for everybody arriving at 7.30! This was so typical of me, however I figured it was yet another funny story to write about in my book. Luckily I had a best friend, Nicola (my guardian angel), who was as a calm as a cucumber as I explained the situation to her on the phone, asked me what needed to be done, and took control of everything, allowing me just to focus on having my last EVER chemotherapy treatment.

When I finally arrived home I actually had time for the quickest dress change in history and a kiss and a cuddle with Lillie before heading off to the cabin, completely in a whirlwind, not really knowing what was going on or having a minute to let it sink in that I had finished chemo.

My friends, Nicola, Hannah and Lynette, had done a great job; the cabin looked great and was ready for the guests to arrive. It was a fabulous evening and I completely let my hair down — or shall we say took my wig off! I'm not sure oncologists would ever advise drinking alcohol one hour after finishing chemo, but I think it's fair to say I had broken every rule that evening. Dave had bought me a bottle of my favourite champagne, Veuve Clicquot. I drank the full bottle — well it was only 100 calories per glass! I also drank ridiculous amounts of prosecco in the hot tub and danced the night away in my still-wet swimming costume. The party finished at around 3am. I remember going to bed feeling exhausted but also happy and content.

The next morning I woke up in bed to find Betty Boobs lying next to me, and my friend, Nicola, on the other side. Betty Boobs was made of balloons and was a replica of me when I had my long hair. I woke feeling very delicate; it was hard to identify whether the effects were from chemo or far too much alcohol! However, what was important was that I had a fabulous time, which made everything so worthwhile. I couldn't have wished for a better way to celebrate my boobs and finishing chemo.

Sunday, 10th May 2015 – The evening before the big op

Feeling nervous as I prepare what I need and packing my case for the hospital – mannequin head and wig being at the top of the priority list! I think making sure I've got everything I need, along with a few home comforts, has helped me to feel more prepared and less anxious. By tomorrow morning it will all be over, my boobs will have gone, taking the big C with them, meaning I have conquered the last part of journey.

A list of hospital essentials:

- Sports bra or front-clasping bra with good support — one size bigger to allow for swelling (remember to ask which bra your surgeon recommends);
- Pyjamas with a button-down top and loose drawstring pants;
- Slippers;
- Lightweight robe;
- Cuddly socks to hide those ugly post-surgery stockings;
- Regular medication — if taking any;
- Make-up;
- Toiletries;
- Baby wipes;
- Lip balm (I used Aloe lips and it was fantastic for keeping my lips moist and I could also use it to rub into my cuticles and nails);
- Ear plugs;
- Books and magazines; and
- Earphones (to listen to your favourite music or relaxation music).

That day before the operation I put the necessary arrangements in place, as I was going to be out of action for at least 10 days. Having such a great husband to hold the fort made everything much easier. That evening, my guardian angel was coming to stay over so that she could be there to look after Lillie. While Nic was there I asked her if she would cast my boobs with a casting kit that my brother had bought for me — as usual I had left it until last minute! Nic said yes but had absolutely no idea what she was letting herself in for.

We decided that the best place to do the deed was in the kitchen and began by pulling out the instructions. I have never seen so my pages of writing! (I don't follow instructions very well.) As it was eleven o'clock at night, we decided to wing it and work out how to do it as we went on. Dave had gone to bed at this point and left us to it. I giggled like a little girl all the way through it and couldn't get over the strange scene of me having my boobs cast by my best friend the eve before my op. It was fair to say our relationship had definitely reached another level of friendship!

As she applied the first wet bandage, I had to try very hard not to let out a squeal from the shock of how cold it was. I have to say she did a great job and the application was easier than what we had both thought…until we got to the nipples! For some reason, even though they were both on show, one of them didn't want to participate! It turned out I had one perfect nipple and one not so perfect. Nicola didn't trust herself to fix it so that it matched the other one, so we left it until the cast was ready to come off. I patched up the misshaped nipple on the cast myself. However, when I had finished I had one normal sized nipple and an extra-large one! Once it was dry I knew that I would be able to sand it down to match them up, but for now it would just have to stay like that. The kitchen table, sink and floor were covered in white dust and blobs of clay! By the time we cleaned up the mess it was one o'clock in the morning. It was time for bed as I had to get my beauty sleep ready for my big op.

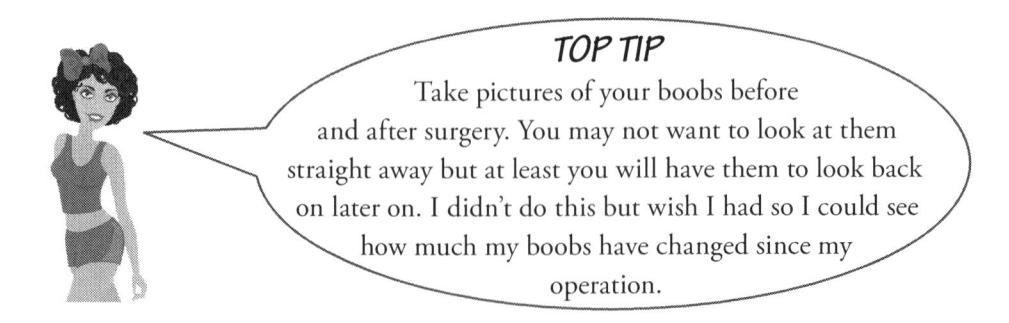

TOP TIP
Take pictures of your boobs before and after surgery. You may not want to look at them straight away but at least you will have them to look back on later on. I didn't do this but wish I had so I could see how much my boobs have changed since my operation.

The next morning Dave and I had to be up at 5.30am to get to Bridgewater hospital in Manchester for 7. On the way there I felt anxious; I knew what was involved with the operation procedure but it was how I was going to feel afterwards that worried me the most.

On the way in we met Dr Mahadev and had a quick chat before he headed off to get ready for surgery. Knowing that he was the surgeon doing my operation gave me the reassurance I needed that I was in safe hands.

When we got to the ward I was taken to my room at the end of the corridor. The first thing I noticed was that it didn't have accessible windows that I could open or have a view of outside, instead they had bars across them because the ward was below ground level. This didn't help my anxiety, as I get a bit claustrophobic in this sort of environment. The room was also quite small; however I was only there for the one night. I got ready and it wasn't long before I had to say goodbye to Dave before being escorted to theatre. The anaesthetist made feel very relaxed and at ease, and I soon drifted off into a beautiful and peaceful sleep.

When I woke, I was in the recovery room. I respond very well to anaesthetic and always wake quite quickly, usually chatting and smiling when I come round (God only knows what I am actually talking about — probably total nonsense). Surgery done, I felt myself become calm and relaxed yet, despite still being drowsy, focused on having some tea and toast — I could smell it as they wheeled me down the corridor! While I was waiting for something to satisfy my grumbling belly, I reflected on my journey, thinking how far I had come from diagnosis and feeling thankful that I had made it this far kicking cancer's butt! After my tea and toast, belly full and feeling very content yet still feeling the fuzzy effects of the anaesthetic, I filmed a video letting everyone know that the operation was successful.

After the op I couldn't see my boobs as they were all bandaged up but I was happy to wait until the bandages were taken off the next day. They felt heavy and I could only see a drainage bottle either side (plastic bottles with a tube that attaches onto the top of it, the other end of the tube is inserted into the breast and then stitched to keep it in position). They were going to be attached to me for the next 10 days. After my refreshments I needed to go to the toilet but needed assistance as I was still a bit drowsy and feeling a bit sore; it was not easy trying to climb out of bed as well as hold on to my drainage bags. I tried to be as dignified as possible but it was quite difficult. Over the next few days it became my focus to master how to move around with them more easily.

TOP TIP
Make sure you pack pyjamas with a button-down top and pants with a drawstring as you will have restricted movement e.g. lifting your arms above shoulder height.

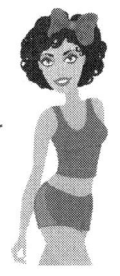

That afternoon Dave and Lillie were coming to visit and I couldn't wait to see them both. Feeling quite exhausted I decided to have a sleep; waking up to find Dave and Lillie at my bedside was the best surprise ever. Dave had brought me a bag full of goodies and it wasn't long before Lillie was tucking into them, sitting on the bed, using my legs to rest on whilst watching Cbeebies. It was such a perfect moment, knowing the operation was over and having my family at my bedside after what we had all been through.

The next day I was being moved to South Cheshire hospital, where I would be spending the next five days. I had really enjoyed my short stay at Bridgewater and the nurses were really lovely, very friendly and consistent. The care I received was excellent and nothing was too much trouble. Dave came to pick me up the next morning. I still hadn't seen my new boobs because I needed to keep the bandages on as extra support whilst travelling.

We arrived at South Cheshire, where I was wheeled down to my ward. All the staff greeted me as I trundled passed, including the chef, who was wearing black trousers, a white shirt, a black bow tie and a black chef's hat. It was the most lovely (yet surreal) hospital experience I had ever had — I felt like a celebrity! My room was perfect; I had plenty of space, a garden view and a window that I could open! The next few days would consist of me resting, relaxing, adjusting to my new boobs and letting my body heal.

The following morning the nurse came to examine me and to empty my drainage bottles — I felt so much lighter. Shortly after, Dr Mahadev came to examine my breasts — it was time for the bandages to come off… eek!

Tuesday, 12th May 2015

The moment of truth… I took a deep breath as the last bandage was removed and looked down. They are completely different to how I imagined them to look! I expected them to be badly bruised and look at lot worse than they did. After Dr Mahadev had left I had a proper inspection of them in the mirror and was surprised to see how good they looked. They are quite swollen so it is difficult to know how they will be in a few days' time when the swelling subsides. They feel very heavy, like big boulders on my chest, and are solid, just like when my boobs were full of milk and ready to explode when I was breastfeeding!

Later that day Dave arrived with the most beautiful bouquet of lilies (my favourite flower, hence why Lillie is called Lillie). He had also brought me some tops that buttoned up at the front. I hadn't realised that after my operation, movement would be restricted, preventing me from being able to get anything over my head. My surgeon had also recommended that I wear a sports bra for support so Dave had to go bra shopping — another first for him! However because of the swelling and me still being quite sore, I wasn't able to fasten the bra. It is common to have swelling and bruising after your operation and is more likely if you have had all the lymph nodes removed. Dave also brought me a bag to transport my drainage bags around more easily. It wasn't the most glamorous bag I have ever used, but it did the job! After doing some research I have since found out about a lady who designs bags specifically to hold drainage bottles. The company is called Drain Dollies. I wish I had of known about these before my op. They are discreet, dignified, really pretty and practical allowing you to make a drink, brush your teeth and move around more easily. A donation from each Drain Dolly sold will go to prevent breast cancer who are investing in new and ongoing research projects to bring us one step closer to a breast cancer free future for all. So, if you don't want to look like a bag lady, have a look at the link in the back of the book!

The next day I wanted to freshen up and clean the two big black arrows and iodine from my skin and also change into some clothes to make me feel more human. I could only manage a wash down with some baby wipes, which got rid of the arrows but only removed a small amount of the yellow iodine. Nevertheless, it did the job and although I wasn't going outside it helped me to feel better mentally.

The swelling started to reduce a few days after the operation, however the bruising came out a lot more, on my left breast especially (this was the breast with the cancer in so I suspect there was more work required with having to also remove the lymph nodes).

Each day I was becoming more self-sufficient, the pain subsided gradually and I didn't have to rely so much on the nurses helping me to wash and change. There was a moment when I was getting changed and I caught a glimpse of myself in the mirror. I didn't recognize the person looking back at me: I had no hair, eyebrows or eyelashes, my skin looked grey, pale and aged and my boobs looked battered and bruised, making me realise just how brutal cancer is. There were many moments like this, when I would feel vulnerable and powerless, wishing that everything had just been a bad dream.

I was determined to make the most of my time left at South Cheshire, ensuring I got as much rest as possible. I had plenty to keep me occupied whilst in hospital, including writing my book and recording a video tutorial to post on my breast cancer page about how to apply eyebrows and eyelashes (which took about five takes because I kept getting interrupted by the nurses). Up until I made the video I hadn't worn make-up, false eyelashes or even pencilled in my eyebrows and had only ever wore my beanie hat since the operation. So, after finishing my tutorial, none of the nurses recognised me and they were totally taken aback by the transformation. They had only ever seen my wig sat on my mannequin head in the bathroom! As one nurse left the room another would appear, wanting to have a look at the newly transformed me.

It became a ritual for me and having to do it every day became the norm; it seemed that when I made myself up, it was like piecing together a jigsaw puzzle which I then took apart at night.

I was inundated with friends and family coming to visit and who spoilt me with my three favourite things: flowers, chocolates and champagne (my room looked and smelt like a florist). I even got my friend, Lindsey, to bring in her hair clippers to remove all of the long wispy bits of hair that had grown back since my op so I didn't look like I had a comb-over! And I really enjoyed my stay at South Cheshire, the nurses were so warm and caring and looked after me so well — even the food was 5* and served silver service style! I couldn't have wished for anything better; it was just what the doctor ordered!

Saturday, 16th May 2015 – Time to go home

I was up bright and early this morning, getting ready and packing my case to go home. I am so excited! As lovely as it has been at South Cheshire, there is no place like home and I am ready to leave. Dave and Lillie aren't coming to pick me up until late morning so I've got plenty of time. Despite feeling excited, there is a part of me that is a bit concerned, knowing I won't have the doctors and nurses on hand, just in case something goes wrong.

Not having people with medical knowledge around when I got home was a worry for me. Although I wasn't anticipating anything going wrong, things do happen. One day at South Cheshire I had an embarrassing moment whilst on the toilet; my tube that was connected via a valve to the tube inside my breast had disconnected. I felt a trickle of warm fluid (which was actually blood) running down my skin as the tube fell to the floor. I panicked, thinking the whole tube had fallen out, and quickly pulled the alarm cord for assistance. A male nurse swiftly came to my aid. Oh no! I had to explain through the door what had happened and then he had to get a female nurse. I managed to get myself off the toilet and cover myself, attempting to keep what bit of dignity I had left. 'Luckily' I had only had a wee, so at least the nurse wouldn't be greeted by any offensive aromas! It wasn't long before the tube was reattached and I was all cleaned up with fresh dressings and good to go, left with another funny story to share in this book!

Before I knew it, it was time to leave. Even though I had only been there for four days, I felt like it was much longer, but in a nice way, and part of me felt sad saying goodbye. Although it wasn't easy trying to hide the tubes attached to my drainage bottles (because they were so long), after a few attempts I managed to secure them under my clothes and looked half decent. On the journey home, Dave asked me if I would like to go for afternoon tea at the local garden centre… of course my answer was YES — I never refuse a cream tea!

When we arrived home I was quite exhausted so I lay on the couch and rested for a little while. Being home was a completely different feeling to how I imagined; I had a mixture of emotions: happy, sad, and apprehensive. When I left home on the morning of my operation, I felt strong and ready to take on the last stage of my journey. For the last five weeks leading up to my op I had started to become independent and felt resilient. However, arriving home this time I felt vulnerable and fragile again, knowing I was now dependant on Dave all over again, like I was when having chemo.

As the days went on I struggled with the fact that I couldn't drive and was limited to what I could do, especially with having the drainage bottles attached to me. When you're in hospital you don't really notice just how immobile you actually are because they have all the necessary facilities. Being at home was a different matter. Sleeping became difficult because I had to have one of the bottles in bed with me because it wasn't possible to hang it over the side of the double bed, so I was always conscious about the blood leaking out…and it's not nice lying next to a bottle of blood, even if it is yours!

The bottles started to become a right pain in the arse. A few days after being home I hit a real low; I'd had enough, mentally and physically. I think my body had taken as much as it could and my boobs didn't feel like they were part of me and were so sore. I was feeling sorry for myself, angry and frustrated that this had happened to me. Dave kept asking me if I was OK and I would say 'yes' because I didn't know how to explain exactly how I was feeling. I needed to be on my own, so I took myself up into the bathroom, locked the door, sat on the floor and sobbed my heart out until I had no more tears left. As I sat there, I thought, 'What am I doing?' The cancer had gone but it was still trying to control me. Once the tears had dried I had a chat with myself, got up off the floor (not so easily) and decided from that moment I would accept there were certain things I couldn't do and find ways of adapting.

For the next six days, I woke up, got dressed and applied a bit of make-up, just to make me feel better mentally. I resolved that, rather than getting frustrated about the fact I couldn't lift or carry anything heavy or drive while the scars healed, I would focus on the things I could do.

Things you can do post-op:

- Folding the washing;
- Making a cup of coffee (only putting a small amount of water in the kettle so you can lift it);
- General tidying (not lifting anything heavy); and
- Preparing food (everything needs to be accessible and below shoulder height to prevent stretching the wounds).

Despite my frustration, the next few days passed quickly and, before I knew it, it was time to say goodbye to my drainage bottles. I was eager to get them out as I was attending a ladies' networking lunch in the day and, that evening, I was having a health, beauty and wellbeing evening to raise money for Macmillan. I was curious to know how they were going to remove the drainage tubes but also a little bit scared about how it would feel and whether it would be painful. Before the tubes could be removed, the dressings under each arm had to be taken off. I couldn't really feel anything because everywhere was numb, but I did notice the hair under my arms had decided to make a miraculous reappearance, which was quite embarrassing! As the stitches were removed, the nurse gently pulled on the tube, which was wrapped around the breast like a spiral. As it unwrapped, it felt like there was a worm wiggling under my skin. It was such a relief once it had been removed. With a fresh dressing on I was good to go. I jumped off the bed and practically skipped out of hospital. I felt so much lighter and I could now drive, so I drove home.

TOP TIP
Most women are ready to drive about four weeks after their operation. Don't drive unless you feel in full control of the car. I starting driving 10 days after my operation.

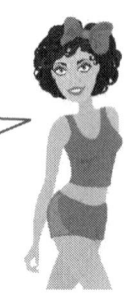

The first thing I did when I got home was to have my first shower in 10 days! I couldn't get the dressing wet, so I couldn't have a complete shower, but I could shower enough of my body to feel clean. After my shower I changed into a short black and cream swing dress, finished off with a red jacket, red lipstick and a pair of black stilettos, before applying my wig that Nicola had kindly blow dried for me — I felt fabulous and was ready to take on the world again! My boobs felt quite squashed in my dress and I still had the sensation that they were about to explode! That aside, it felt so good to be out on my own, driving, feeling like me again!

On the Saturday I decided to go bra shopping as I only had the one bra that Dave had got for me, which still wouldn't fasten properly at the back. It had been great as a temporary measure until I was able to go shopping myself and I couldn't wait to choose my own. I decided to go to M&S as I'd had bras from there before and they were always good quality. It didn't take long choosing a bra as I was just looking at the sports bras, which only come in a minimal selection. As I got to the changing room, I asked the lady if she could assist me and explained the reasons why. She couldn't do enough for me, especially when I asked her if I could remove my wig because it was so hot in the changing room. (Since my op, my hair has started growing very quickly, especially on my head and face!) I showed her the bras I wanted to try on but explained I wasn't really sure what size I was as a 32DD was too small. She went away, bringing back a 34DD and 36DD. The 34DD was too tight and the 36DD fitted perfectly — flipping heck, my boobs were much bigger than I thought! (See, this is why a catalogue of boobs would be a great idea!) Fitting done, I left M&S feeling very supported and comfortable in my new bra.

The following week I went back to see Dr Mahadev so he could examine my new boobs and see how they were healing. He was very happy with their progress, which meant I could have the last remaining dressings removed. For the next two weeks I would have weekly appointments and then, after that, they would be spread out so I would have an appointment after one month, then three months and then, finally, after six months.

I had asked my surgeon what I could do to speed up the healing process and to help strengthen my upper torso. He recommended yoga, so I looked for a yoga class locally and found a fantastic yoga teacher, Kate Marshall (website can be found at the back of the book). Kate was very sympathetic and understanding of my situation and advised me on which yoga movements I could and couldn't do. I started yoga with Kate six weeks after my op, attending one session per week, and it has made a massive difference to my core and upper body strength. I am still attending 12 months on and have met some other ladies at the class who have also had breast surgery and have now become my friends. I also had six months of MLD — Manual Lymphatic Drainage — due to some swelling from the lymph node removal. This also sped up my recovery and allowed me to regain full use of my arm much more quickly, enabling me to get on with day-to-day daily chores.

> **TOP TIP**
> After a mastectomy or having lymph nodes removed, your shoulder or arm may feel sore or stiff. It's important to do the arm exercises. This will help improve your movement and reduce the risk of long-term problems. Start the exercises as soon as you can.

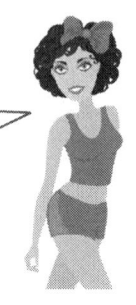

The next few pages show some of the exercises that helped me after surgery. You should do the exercises every day. It is recommended to do them morning, midday and evening. However, sometimes this can be difficult and it depends on how you are feeling, so always do what feels right for you and listen to what your body is telling you. You should feel stretching and pulling when you exercise but it shouldn't be painful.

*Go to **www.sarahsstory.co.uk** to download your free step by step exercise video.*

POST-SURGERY EXERCISES
Level 1 exercises

Pendula exercise
- Relax your arm and let it hang down, gently.
- Do it for 1-2 minutes and repeat 3-4 times per day.

Shoulder circling
- Keep your arms loose and relaxed by your sides.
- Shrug your shoulders up and towards your ears, then circle them back down.

Rotating the arms out to the side
- Stand upright and keep your arm into the side with 90° bent elbows and rotate your arm as far as you can.
- Be gentle — no forcing.
- Repeat 10 times, up to 3-4 times per day.

Sliding towel up the wall
- Stand in front of the wall.
- Have a rolled up towel in your hands.
- Keep your arms close to your body.
- Slide the towel up the wall with both hands as far as you can and slowly back down again.
- Repeat up to 10 times, 2-3 times per day.
-

Bouncing the ball
- Hold a small ball (a children's toy ball is ideal).
- Bounce the ball several times for 1-2 minutes until the arm gets tired.
- Repeat 2 times per day.

Sliding the ball up the wall
- Hold a small ball and face the wall.
- Do circles with the ball on the wall and slowly move it up as far as you can and slowly down again.
- Repeat 3 times, 2 times per day.

Squeezing the shoulder blades together
- Stand upright and have your elbows bent at 90° close to your body.
- Try to squeeze your shoulder blades together.
- Repeat 10 times, 3-4 times per day.

Level 2 exercises

External rotating of the arm lying down

- Lie on your back with your knees bent up.
- Put your affected arm out 30° from your body and have your elbow bent in 90°.
- Put a towel underneath your arm so your arm is level with your body.
- Slowly rotate your arm outwards as far as you can and back up into neutral.
- It is important that you don't force the arm into position.
- Repeat 10 times and up to 3 sets with 10 repetitions.

Squeezing the shoulder blades together with a resistance band

- Stand facing the wall.
- Put a theraband/resistance band around the door handle.
- Bend elbow to 90° degrees and pull the band so that you feel that you are squeezing the shoulder blades together.
- Repeat 3 sets with 10 repetitions.

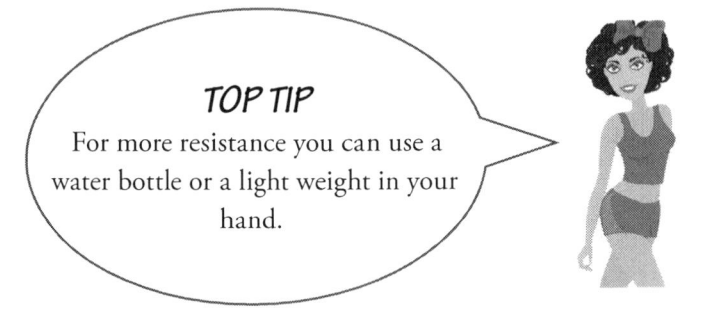

TOP TIP
For more resistance you can use a water bottle or a light weight in your hand.

Level 3 exercises

Rotator cuff exercise with arm elevation and stepping forward
- Stand upright.
- Keep your arms close to your body with your arm and elbows bent to 90°.
- Put the theraband/ resistance band in a loop around your hands and push gently into the band.
- Keep the resistance on the theraband/ resistance band whilst your raise your arms to the ceiling and slowly bring them back down.
- At the same time as you raise your arms take a step forward and when your arms come back down then step back again.
- Repeat up to 5-8 times and gradually work up to 2 sets of 10 repetitions.

Progression of same exercise
- Instead of stepping forward you can step up on a step and back down again whilst your elevate your arms to the ceiling with the theraband band/ resistance band OR
- Stand against the wall with a pilates ball and keep your legs a little bit away from the wall and do squats and elevate your arms with the theraband/ resistance band at the same time.
- Repeat 10 times and gradually work up to 2 sets of 10 repetitions.

> **TOP TIPS**
> - All exercises should be pain free.
> - Don't do any of the exercises if you are not sure how to perform them.
> - Don't force your shoulders.
> - Do all the exercises gently.
> - If you feel uncomfortable with any of the exercises whilst doing them, stop immediately.

By doing the exercises my breasts were settling much quicker and I no longer felt like I had two big boulders pressing against my chest. They still felt heavy and 'extra-large' but nothing like when I first had my operation.

One thing I had noticed was that every now and again my arm would make an embarrassing farting noise…luckily never when I was in public! When I was in school I remember boys putting their hand under their arm and moving the arm up and down, creating a vacuum, which made a farting noise. I couldn't do this at the time (nor did I want to) but now I can make this sound without even having to use my hands! It doesn't happen on my right breast, however it happens on the breast that had the cancer. I think it's because the implant on my left side is positioned differently and protrudes more than the other side, creating the noise when my arm brushes against it. So, post op I have been left with a farty arm! And post chemo, I was left with a furry face — beautiful!

Three months after my op and Dave, Lillie and I went to Greece for a well-deserved family holiday. Due to my scars still being fresh and still having to wear a sports bra, I decided not to go bikini shopping but to wear a swimming costume that I bought when I had my Boob Voyage party. It wasn't a perfect fit, but it covered the majority of my boobs, including my scars.

Saturday, 15th August 2015 – Visiting Fiskardo

Today we visited a Greek fishing village called Fiskardo, which has a gorgeous bay where you can go for a swim. What a beautiful place! It has been an extremely hot day and I was desperate to go into that crystal-clear water so I decided I would go to the shop and have a look at some bikinis. I started by looking at the less expensive selections and picked out a couple that I liked and took them into the changing room, feeling a bit anxious about how they were going to look and how I was going to feel, knowing my scars would be on show for everybody to see. I tried on the first style, a pretty design with no padding in the cups, which I didn't feel I would need due to the size of my new boobs. It didn't look at all right and made my boobs look flat. My second choice was a halter neck with a padded cup. This one made my boobs look shapelier but it still didn't look right – in fact, I didn't like what I saw. Although I feel so blessed and thankful to be alive and know that having a double mastectomy has given a better chance of surviving, I can't help but feel sad.

Looking in the mirror, I saw myself standing there with my short hair and fashioning my new 'breast cancer' boobs (which don't look anything like the way they do when you have a boob job – they look flat and misshapen, with scars which are a constant reminder of what you have just been through). After 30 minutes I decided to go with the padded bra (which Dave said I looked great in). However, despite being 50 euros out of pocket and still not convinced with my purchase, I felt happy that I could now enjoy a swim in the sea with Dave and Lillie. As we approached the bay I found myself starting to feel self-conscious about how I looked in my new bikini and paranoid about the fact people will probably think my scars are from having a boob job and not the fact I have just had a double mastectomy from having breast cancer. The people were probably not paying any attention to me but I couldn't help feeling a little embarrassed. The walk from where we sat to the sea felt like miles and it seemed like a lifetime before I actually reached the water. As the cold salt water touched my feet, I began to relax and immersed my body into the water, enjoying the fact Dave, Lillie and I are together, having such a fantastic holiday in such a beautiful place.

People assume that having a mastectomy is the same as having a boob job but it's nothing like it, it's completely different because they take away all your breast tissue and, in some cases, you can no longer breastfeed. You also have reconstructive surgery, where they then MAY have to take muscle skin grafts from your back or thighs, meaning more scaring and wounds that can sometimes become infected. Before having my op, I had imagined in my mind how my new boobs would look and couldn't wait to show them off in my new bras and bikinis. However, reality was nothing as I had imagined. I couldn't help but feel disappointed and disillusioned by the result.

Since my op eight months ago, I have been wearing sports bras to give my boobs the support they need after surgery. However, although they are brilliant for support and the healing process, they are not pretty, very bland and don't make you feel womanly or sexy!

Whilst on the web I decided to look at what bargains H&M had in their sale. I came across two beautiful lace bras, one in red and one in black, and decided to order them in the hope that they would fit. I waited eagerly for my new lingerie to arrive. A few days later my new bras finally landed on the doormat. I couldn't wait to unwrap them and the excitement was like Christmas as a child all over again — plastic wrapping thrown everywhere! When I finally got them out of the packaging they were as beautiful as they looked on the internet — I couldn't wait to try them on. I undid the clasps of my favourite — a lovely hot red lace — and positioned the bra, hoping it was the perfect fit. I fastened the clasp with great difficulty, breathing in, in some hope this would make a difference as it was too tight. Once it was fastened I arranged my boobs within the cups, again, with some effort. Nevertheless, still in denial that it would fit, I adjusted the straps and, in excited anticipation, looked in the mirror. To my major disappointment it looked hideous — the cups only covered around my areola and, as soon as I allowed myself to relax and breathe, the bra squashed very tightly against my breastbone and the strap pinched under my arm. In my frustration I threw the rest back into the packaging, too disheartened to try any others on. My first online bra shopping experience was a complete disaster! So what I have learnt?

- *Having a mastectomy is not like having a boob job. WHY? Because your boobs are flatter and not as pert!*
- *Mastectomy boobs are a weird shape and not true to a 'normal' fake boob size!*
- *I can no longer get cheap bras in the sale via the internet. From now on I need to go into a specialist shop to be sized correctly and pay full price — see you in Rigby and Peller!*

> ***While your boobs are still healing you will need bras with:***
>
> - soft seams;
> - a wide underband;
> - fully adjustable straps;
> - full cups;
> - minimal detailing; and
> - underwires.

I've since realized that the type of bra you will need after surgery will change. You will find your boobs will change a few months after surgery and will keep changing as time goes on. My boobs are completely different to how they looked 12 months ago. This can also depend on your diet and how your body changes over time.

> **TOP TIP**
> Whether you have had a reconstruction or use a prosthesis, avoid wearing an underwired bra until the area has healed from surgery as the wires can apply pressure to an implant and affect how a prosthesis sits.

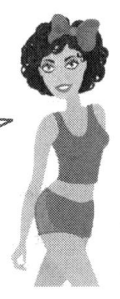

Even shopping for clothes has become complicated because of my bust size. When choosing clothes (especially anything that buttons or that zips up at the front), they don't fit the same. Before I had my operation, I had always been a size 10 top and bottom, however, post op, I'm having to buy a size 12, sometimes bigger depending on the style. My most recent buy was a coat. I had ordered a size 10, but when it came it was way too tight around my boobs although it fitted perfectly around my waist. I sent it back and got a 12 and it fitted better around the bust but was a bit big around the waist (it had a belt so I was able to get away with it). I also have to be careful wearing tight tops as they don't look very flattering, especially when wearing a sports bra, because they make my boobs look really flat and huge. At no point on the build-up to my operation had I taken fashion disasters into account! Since then I have become aware of companies such as 'Bravissimo' and 'Pepperberry' that do clothes and lingerie with different bust sizes but still have small waist sizes. (websites for both are available in the back of the book)

In the months after a mastectomy my body is still continuing to adjust to the effects of the surgery. I had sharp shooting pains in both my breasts for a couple of months after my operation but they eventually subsided. My Macmillan nurse warned me that I may have strange sensations or pains in the months after as the nerves regrow, such as a sharp shooting or stabbing pain, or a throbbing, aching or oppressing pain. The discomfort can go away by itself, or it can persist but you do adapt. It's over a year since my operation and I still get twinges every now and again and a dull ache on the side where they removed all my lymph nodes. I notice it becomes much worse if I don't exercise.

I've recently been to see my oncologist because my implants have changed shape and one of my breasts became sore, which they believed could be to do with the implant. This can be a long-term problem after implant surgery. Although silicone is safe, it is still foreign to the body. The normal reaction of the body to any foreign tissue is to form a fibrous covering around it. The fibrous covering is known as a capsule. Over the years, the capsule can shrink, squeezing the implant. Doctors call this 'capsular contracture' and it happens in about 1 in 6 patients. It makes the breast painful and hard, and changes its shape. If the shape changes a lot, you may have to have the implant taken out and replaced. The shape of my breast has changed drastically and the pain has gone, however, I have two different sized boobs (which may be connected to a change in weight — I lost weight then have put weight back on since my operation). My options are to learn to live with what I have got or to go under the knife again to put things right. However, there is no guarantee that nothing will go wrong again in the future. I'd be putting my body through more stress and anxiety — maybe for no benefit. Maybe just purchasing a very good push up bra with extra padding will do the job! I'm still yet to decide but I think the bra option is the favourite to win at the moment.

Although I don't plan to get secondary cancer, you can never say never! Twelve months after treatment I was feeling tired all the time, suffering from headaches, as well as feeling breathless and experiencing abdominal pain. I went to my GP and reported it to my Macmillan nurse. The GP examined me and asked to see me the following week. Within that week I noticed my breast had become sore and I could feel a lump. It was the opposite breast to where they found the cancer. I couldn't believe it and my head went into a complete spin — not again! I just couldn't face another round of everything I had been through. I went back to my GP straight away and had a secondary examination. The GP confirmed there was a lump and an appointment was made to see my surgeon. I cried all the way to the hospital, terrified it had come back to get me a second time. She referred me for an ultrasound as she thought there may still be tissue in the breast from my operation. Thankfully it was all clear. I didn't know the symptoms of secondary cancer at this point and it's difficult to know sometimes whether things like tiredness and loss of appetite are still the effects of chemotherapy.

I want to share the symptoms with you so you can act quickly and report them if you experience any from the list.

Symptoms of secondary cancer:

- Pain in the back or hips that does not improve with pain relief;
- Feeling constantly tired;
- Ongoing headache;
- A constant feeling of nausea;
- A dry cough or feeling breathless; and
- Unexplained weight loss and loss of appetite.

Having got over my scare, I am starting to fall in love with my boobs all over again. OK, they are not my original boobs and OK, one is still a different shape and size to the other, but I am learning how to dress myself to look good all over again, keeping up with my exercises and hey, what a fantastic excuse to have to buy expensive lingerie!

CHAPTER EIGHT

Giving Myself The Best Chance

Throughout my journey I knew it was very important to do everything I could possible to give me the best chance of beating breast cancer. After my diagnosis I had absolutely no idea how I was going to do this, so I sat myself down and had a think about my plan of action.

I came up with a list of five areas of my life where small adjustments could make all the difference:

- *Diet & nutrition;*
- *Fitness;*
- *Holistic therapies;*
- *Looking good; and*
- *Family and friends.*

Diet and Nutrition

We all know that diet and nutrition is good for your health, even if you don't have an illness. However, I didn't realise just how important it would be to my recovery. After my diagnosis I had a meeting with my Macmillan nurse, who informed me of a study called B-AHEAD 2. It was a diet being carried out by Wythenshawe Hospital in Manchester and had come to national attention when the doctor and journalist Michael Mosley adapted it in his 'the fast diet' book in January 2013. A month later, BBC journalist Kate Harrison published her version — 'The 5:2 diet book'. Although all three diets vary slightly, they all have the same general principle.

Dr Michelle Harvie and Professor Tony Howell of Prevent Breast Cancer (based at Wythenshawe hospital) were testing whether having a specific diet would have a positive effect on breast cancer patients having chemotherapy. At this point this was the only information I had, however, I definitely knew I wanted to be part of the study.

Following on from the meeting with my Macmillan nurse, I attended a literary lunch where I met Dr Michelle Harvie, who was talking about her 'The 2–day diet'. Having not heard about the diet previously to being told about it twice in a matter of days was quite a coincidence – it was a sign! I was intrigued by how two days per week of low calories and low carbohydrates can be effective for weight loss and reducing levels of insulin, a hormone that is linked to the risk of breast cancer and other common diseases such as diabetes and heart disease. The lunch happened the day after my lymph node biopsy so I was still in a bit of a daze but I knew I wanted to do everything I could to keep healthy.

After Dr Harvie finished her talk, I plucked up the courage to talk to her. To be honest, it wasn't that difficult as she was lovely to speak to, so I told her that my Macmillan nurse had informed me about the diet the previous week and I was very keen to be involved in the study. She was eager for me to take part as I was a young patient, so I gave my details to be passed on to the research team who would call me the following week. That evening when I got home I did a bit research to find out a bit more about the diet and this is what I found:

> The B-AHEAD 2 research study is testing whether a new intermittent diet can be better than a standard daily healthy eating diet in 170 women who are having chemotherapy after surgery for breast cancer. Half of the women who decide to take part in the study will followed this new diet which involves a low carbohydrate and low calorie diet for two days per week, and half will followed a daily calorie controlled diet. Both groups are also advised to undertake 150 minutes of moderate exercise per week.
>
> The study investigates how easy these two diets are to follow during chemotherapy, if they help to reduce the side effects of chemotherapy and which is better for controlling weight. They will recruit 170 patients from the University Hospital South Manchester and 10 other breast cancer centres in Greater Manchester and Cheshire. Throughout the participants' course of chemotherapy, their weight, body fat and muscle mass, blood levels, hormones and inflammation linked to the risk of recurrence, side effects from chemotherapy and their well-being will be assessed.
>
> preventbreastcancer.org.uk

A week later I received a call from the research team and a date was arranged for my appointment to start the program. As part of the study I would be given advice on diet and exercise, but first they needed to assess my current diet patterns. Therefore I needed to complete a 7-day food diary, sticking to my usual diet and activity routines, therefore providing them with better information in order for them to give the correct advice and guidance.

On the day of my appointment I met a researcher who took details of my medical and family history, including planned breast cancer treatments. I then had a blood test — this meant no eating or drinking (except water) for 12 hours prior to appointment as this can affect the accuracy of the tests. It was also advised not to have alcohol, eat fish oil or exercise for 24 hours before.

After the blood test I was given a complimentary 'light' breakfast at the Genesis Café —toast and decaffeinated tea or coffee. After my breakfast I had a DXA scan, a simple scan that measures your body fat and your bone density. The scan looks at where you store fat and does not detect cancer. After this my blood pressure was taken as well as my weight and body measurements. They also assessed my fitness by making me walk on a treadmill. Once the assessment was complete I was then informed as to which diet group I had been randomly assigned to and was given my detailed, personalised diet and exercise advice. I was allocated to do the 2-day diet. This involved having two 'restricted' days a week when I would restrict my carbohydrate intake, and the other five days would be 'unrestricted', when I would follow a healthy balanced diet.

I was given a booklet explaining the diet. It described the benefits of a Mediterranean diet, which is high in wholegrains and uses more monounsaturated fats (olives, olive and rapeseed oil, avocados, peanuts, pistachios) and less saturated fat (fatty red processed meats [for example, lamb, pork, duck, sausages and corned beef], palm oil, chocolate and high fatty dairy foods such as cream, full cream, milk, cheese and butter). Also, including fruits, vegetables and oily fish in your diet can benefit your heart as well as decrease the risk of breast cancer recurrence.

Generally to lose weight we either need to cut down our food intake or increase our physical activity levels, or ideally do a combination of both. However, unfortunately chemotherapy can cause a small decrease in your metabolic rate, meaning your body needs less energy than it did before treatment started. This is one of the reasons why many women put on weight when going through chemotherapy for breast cancer. Other reasons for weight gain are that women become less active during chemotherapy and comfort eat after being put on a short course of steroids, which increases appetite.

The 2-day diet included two restricted low carbohydrate days ('restricted' days) each week. We were advised to do these together each week and before chemotherapy. I was required to record these days on my study calendar. The two low carb days are quite similar to the Atkins diet, however, the 2-day diet, in my opinion, was a healthier version, ensuring you have a range of healthy protein foods, the right balance of healthy fats and allows you to have some fruit and vegetables.

> *Examples of foods you can have on a restricted day:*
>
> - Protein foods;
> - Healthy fats;
> - 3 dairy portions;
> - 1 portion of low carb fruit;
> - 5 portions of low carb vegetables or salad;
> - At least 2 litres of low calorie drinks.

Each of these were explained in more detail in the booklets I was given by the research team. There were a variety of booklets: meal ideas and recipes for the 2 days, my guide to the 2-day diet, and ways to keep active through chemotherapy. Reading and familiarising myself with as much information as possible helped give me a better understanding of the foods I should and should not be eating. I took a daily diary of the foods I had eaten throughout the day, which helped me to keep track of what I was eating and allowed me to monitor my portions, making sure I was sticking to my daily allocated amount, as well as giving me something to focus on and keep my brain active!

A couple of my favorite snack recipes for my 'restricted' days were broccoli soup and garlicky balsamic mushrooms and, for my mains, lemon chicken and a lovely shepherd's pie with cauliflower topping. They were all so delicious and easy to make. I especially liked the idea of swapping the shepherd's pie topping to cauliflower instead of potato. It was also food that suited the rest of my family so I didn't have to cook something special just for me. For my 'unrestricted' days, carrot and red lentil soup, fish pie and vegetable rainbow chilli were just a few of the delicious recipes I had to choose from. Each recipe was easy to follow and listed the portions per serving and preparation time.

Here are examples of what I ate on a restricted and unrestricted day:

RESTRICTED DAY

Breakfast
- 2 boiled eggs
- Smoothie made with 7 strawberries, 3 tablespoons of low fat yoghurt and 100 ml semi-skimmed milk

Lunch
- Prawn salad
  7 prawns
- 2 garlic cloves
- Handful of mixed leaf salad
- 6 cherry tomatoes
- ½ inch cucumber
- 30g feta cheese
- 2 slices of red onion
- ½ avocado

Dinner
- Small piece of salmon fillet
- Handful of spinach
- 2 florets of broccoli

Drinks
- 4 glasses of water
- 1 cappuccino
- 1 lime juice of sugar-free cordial and soda water
- Hot chocolate with 10ml of semi-skimmed milk

> **NON-RESTRICTED DAY**
>
> *Breakfast*
> - 1 slice of wholemeal toast
> - Scraping of Bertolli butter and lemon curd
>
> *Lunch*
> - Carrot and lentil soup
>   - Chicken stock
>   - 8 carrots
>   - 50g lentils
> - Small pot of fruit
>   - Pineapple
>   - Melon
>   - Strawberries
>   - Grapes
> - Fat free Strawberry Muller Light yoghurt (small pot)
>
> *Dinner*
> - Cod in breadcrumbs
> - 4 baby potatoes
> - Handful of peas and sweetcorn
> - 6 green beans
> - 4 carrot batons
> - 3 florets of broccoli
> - 2tbls spoons of sour cream
>
> Drinks
> - 1.5 litres water

The diet helped educate me in what type of foods I should be eating, not only whilst going through chemo, but in day-to-day life. Throughout the diet, just like with the medical process, I became like a sponge, absorbing every bit of information. I found it so interesting and realised just how important food is and the negative impact it can have on our lives if we don't put the right food in our bodies.

It is so easy to make small changes such as changing pasta and bread to wholegrain varieties, which have more fibre and nutrients in them compared to white versions and take longer to digest and absorb, keeping you full for longer. One thing I found really interesting was that refined carbohydrates and sugary foods can cause the body to produce lots of insulin, which is not good as insulin can promote the development of cancer growth. It is much better to have a meal consisting of protein and vegetables before eating a cake or eating sweets as it fills you up, releasing the insulin at a much slower rate than if you were to have a meal high in carbohydrates (for example, a pizza or white pasta), leaving you feeling hungry and releasing the insulin much more quickly. This was something I used to do quite a lot on weekends before my diagnosis. However, now I will always make sure I have a low carb meal consisting of salad, vegetables and protein (if I do have pasta, it will be wholemeal) before I allow any treats to pass my lips!

The diet allowed me to understand that the two main types of polyunsaturated fats — omega-3 and omega-6 — are both needed in our diets. Omega-3 fats are particularly good for the heart. Most people eat too much omega-6, which results in the omega-3 not being able to do its job properly. We need to make sure our bodies are getting more omega-3. Below is a table of the foods rich in omega-3 that we need to eat more of and those high in omega-6 that we need to eat less of.

Omega-3 foods *(try to eat more of these)*	*Omega-6 foods* *(try to eat less of these)*
• Oily fish* — fresh or tinned (if tinned, in water or brine) • Fish oil capsules • Walnuts • Rapeseed and soya oil • Flaxseed (also known as linseed) oil and capsules • Omega-3 eggs	• Sunflower seeds and oil • Sunflower margarine • Tinned fish in sunflower oil • Corn oil • Sesame seeds and oil • Chicken skin • Pine nuts

* Fish that are rich in omega-3 are sardines, mackerel, fresh tuna, salmon, herring, pilchards and trout.

A study carried out by researchers from the University of Washington and the University of California followed just over 35,000 postmenopausal women for up to seven years to investigate how their use of supplements, including fish oil, affected their risk of developing breast cancer.[1] It found that the women using fish oil supplements reduced the risk of developing ductal carcinoma, the most common type of breast cancer. However, it also stated that further research is needed. Another study by researchers from Fox Chase Cancer Center reported that omega–3 fatty acids stop or slow the proliferation of all types of cancerous cells, but particularly triple negative breast cancer cells.[2] Proliferation in those types of cells was reduced by as much as 90 per cent.

---

[1] http://www.nhs.uk/news/2010/July07/Pages/omega-3-fish-oil%20may-breast-cancer.aspx
[2] https://www.foxchase.org/news/2013-04-09-omega-3-fatty-acids-breast-cancer

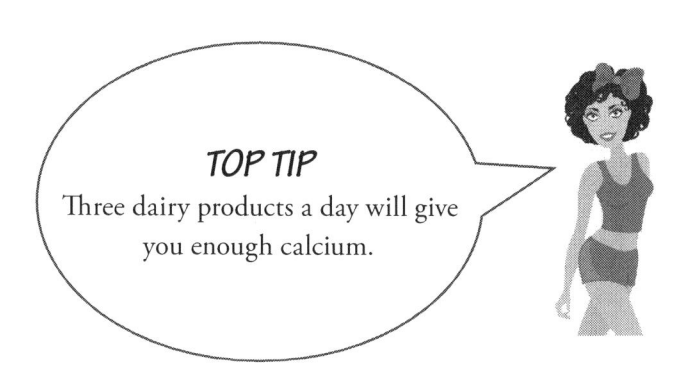

> **TOP TIP**
> Three dairy products a day will give you enough calcium.

Calcium was another important part of my diet as it strengthens bones. Research also suggests that adequate calcium intake may ward off colorectal, ovarian and breast cancers. It is recommended that you can get your calcium intake through a variety of foods.

Foods rich in calcium

- Milk (semi-skimmed or skimmed);
- Alternative 'milks' with added calcium, e.g. soya, nut, oat (sweetened or unsweetened);
- Reduced fat evaporated milk;
- Yoghurt: diet fruit, fat free, low fat;
- Greek and fromage frais, low fat, plain, plain soya yoghurt;
- Cottage cheese;
- Cream cheese (light or extra light);
- Quark; and
- Lower fat cheeses made with pasteurised milk: reduced fat cheddar, Edam, ricotta, mozzarella.

The diet helped me to understand that low fat dairy products are an important source of calcium and contain just as much as their full fat equivalents, but with less of the harmful saturated fats.

It's also important to make sure your vegetable intake is more than your fruit intake. I used to think I was being good by having five portions of fruit a day, however it is much better to have only have two portions of fruit and five or more portions of vegetables as they have fewer calories. Green vegetables such as broccoli, cabbage, kale and Brussels sprouts contain fibre, which eliminates toxins. Broccoli also contains indoles, and especially indol-3-carbinol, which might protect against oestrogen-driven cancers like some breast, prostate, brain and colorectal cancers. Too much fruit can cause you to put on more weight because of the hidden sugars naturally present. There is no evidence that having lots of extra fruit will help your recovery or reduce the risk of breast cancer recurrence; however the weight gain it can cause is not good for your health.

There are many high-risk foods that you have to be aware of because your body is more susceptible to infections during chemotherapy.

High risk foods (Avoid)	*Alternative foods*
• Raw or uncooked meat, poultry, fish (e.g. sushi) and shellfish • Smoked meats, e.g. salami, chorizo, Parma ham, serrano ham • Pâté sold in the refrigerated section of the supermarkets • Taramasalata	• Meat, poultry, fish and shellfish (fresh or frozen) should be thoroughly cooked through (to about 70°C). • Tinned fish and meat • Vacuum-packed, refrigerated meat and poultry • Vacuum-packed, refrigerated fish, including smoked salmon eaten straight from a new packet
• Unpasteurised or mould-ripened soft cheeses such as feta, goats cheese, brie, camembert and blue cheeses (e.g. Roquefort, Danish blue)	• Cheeses, hard or soft, made with pasteurised milk e.g. cheddar, Edam, cream cheese • Look for versions of feta made from pasteurised milk
• 'Bio' or 'probiotic' yoghurts or those containing added bacteria (e.g. Yakult, Activia, Actimel) • Yoghurt made from unpasteurised milk • Unpasteurised cream / milk	• Any other yoghurt e.g. live yoghurt • Pasteurised milk or cream
• Raw or partially cooked eggs or products containing uncooked egg e.g. homemade ice cream and mayonnaise, mousse, hollandaise sauce	• Fully cooked eggs • Shop bought mayonnaise or ice-cream • Other products made with pasteurised eggs

Extract from the 2-day diet book

Sometimes I found it difficult not being able to eat certain high-risk food (such as goat's cheese, feta, blue cheese, salami, chorizo and pâté) and it was not easy at first having to adapt to a brand new of eating. Shopping took more time as I would need to read the labels for the ingredients and for a while I had to carry my booklet around to help guide me in the right direction.

Another thing I struggled with was only being able to have 150 calories of treats, limiting me to a maximum of three treats a week, for example: a two-fingered KitKat, ice cream (2 standard scoops), 5 small squares of chocolate or a 25g bag of crisps. Now, for some people this may be an adequate amount, but for someone who ate a 100g bar of chocolate most weekends and did not think twice about eating her way through a 200g bag of Doritos, this was challenging!

I also found it difficult not being able to have a glass of wine; having said that, my taste buds had changed so much with chemo that wine tasted very metallic. Also, it is 240 calories per glass and counts as 3.3 units per glass, and I was only allowed less than 10 units per week on my diet. Fizzy drinks were more attractive. Before having chemo I very rarely drank fizzy drinks because I've always preferred water. However, I was allowed fizzy drinks as long as they were sugar free. I became very fond of lime cordial and soda water with a slice of fresh lime and crushed ice; it was the only drink that helped me to feel better when I was feeling really nauseous. It tastes delicious and is so thirst quenching, I don't know what it is but the bubbles taste really good. Another drink I really enjoyed when I wasn't feeling sick was prosecco… however, when I read in my booklet that Champagne was only 100 calories and 1.5 of my units, it made much more sense to be a Champagne girl through chemo! Most of the time I didn't really want to drink anything else but water or lime cordial and soda water but it was nice to know I could have alcohol whenever I felt like it as long as it was within my weekly amount.

There would be some days when I didn't feel hungry but I still tried to stick to my diet the best I could. I would always make sure I had breakfast, as this is the most important meal of the day, even if I could only manage a piece of wholemeal toast on my unrestricted days and one egg on restricted days. An egg with a pinch of salt was great to help stop nausea. For the rest of the day I would just snack on foods that were suitable for restricted and unrestricted days.

> ### *Snack suggestions for restricted and unrestricted days*
> - Cooked vegetables with cottage cheese or low-fat hummus;
> - Celery sticks filled with low-fat cheese;
> - Fruit;
> - Bowl of soup;
> - Avocado, mozzarella, tomato and basil stacks;
> - Small handful of nuts (for example, pistachios, brazil or walnuts);
> - Yoghurt;
> - Smoothie made with skimmed or semi-skimmed milk, yoghurt and one piece of fruit; and
> - Sugar free jelly.

An unfortunate side effect of the steroids would be constipation, which would last 2-3 days; I found by increasing my water intake, drinking 100% inner leaf aloe vera gel, getting some gentle exercise and eating more fibre (i.e. more fruit, vegetable, beans, pulses, lentils, high fibre breakfast cereals, whole grain bread, pasta and rice) really helped stop the constipation.

Taking part in the diet definitely contributed to keeping my weight down, helped me feel less bloated and more energized, and made me feel alert and focused. Each week throughout chemo my weight would be taken and recorded and it would only ever increase by two or three pounds and maybe decrease the following week by a pound or two. By the time I finished the diet (which was four months after I finished chemo), my weight was the lowest it had ever been but was still a healthy weight for my height. Also, after repeating the fitness test carried out at the beginning of the study, they found that my fitness levels had pretty much stayed the same (however, I do feel this is because of how active I was during treatment, which I will say more about further on in the chapter). Not only did the diet have a positive impact on my weight but also on me mentally; it kept my mind active, allowing me to focus on something other than chemo. It actually made chemo days more enjoyable because, having two low carb restricted days before chemo day made me look forward to having a sandwich, Starbucks coffee and a treat!

Even though I no longer have to continue to follow the diet plan, I still do but on a much more relaxed basis. I now alternate my no carbs days (restricted) to suit my diary of events and have a few more treats and units of alcohol. The downside is that I no longer have the excuse to drink Champagne, apart from on special occasions, so it generally tends to be wine and prosecco — which isn't too bad! Continuing with the diet and making sure I get the necessary foods needed to keep me at optimum health is very important.

I believe that taking certain supplements such as Royal Jelly, Fish Oils (fish and calamari oil) and an Aloe Vera drink (100% inner leaf) helped support my health in a positive way during treatment. I had been using these products prior to my diagnosis and was determined to continue to take them during treatment. However, it was something I had to discuss with my oncologist. I knew that the Aloe Vera drink may help to keep my immune system strong, my bowel movements functioning at an optimised level and also could help boost my energy levels. I did some research into the benefits of royal jelly and found out that there are claims that it helps with insomnia — which I knew was a major side effect of the steroids. Fish Oils including omega-3 and omega-9 were highly recommended to help reduce heart problems, but also, after doing some research, there are claims it can have a positive on reducing cancerous cells, especially triple negative cancers.

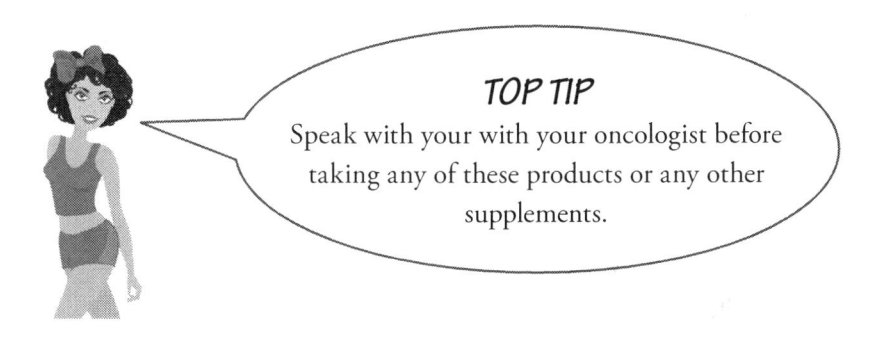

> **TOP TIP**
> Speak with your with your oncologist before taking any of these products or any other supplements.

Exercise

Exercising was something I had always really enjoyed and a few months before my diagnosis I had taken up running. I ran three times a week whenever possible and had taken part in a couple of trail running events. I would generally run three-and-a-half miles, but as much as six miles and more whenever I could. It wasn't easy and I had to work my way up to being able to run comfortably without stopping. Running gave me a release and helped me to decompress, especially if I had had a challenging day.

Leading up to my diagnosis I had been running more as I was training for a 13-mile trail event called 'Hellrunner', which was going to be the longest distance I had ever done! The day I received my diagnosis, after the initial shock when I came home,

I said to Dave I needed to go for a run so I went upstairs, jumped into my running gear, put on my trainers and went for a three-mile run. Receiving the news felt so surreal and, as I was running, I kept playing what the surgeon had said over and over again in my head. All I kept thinking was how we were going to tell Lillie and break the news to my family. Going for a run allowed me some time on my own to gather my thoughts and work out how I was going to get through the next 12 months. Something that became clear whilst I was on the run was that the symptoms of fatigue and pain I had been experiencing prior to my diagnosis were signs of having cancer.

Running became an important part of my daily routine in the early stages of diagnosis. It not only helped me to deal with everything that was going on but also made me more aware that keeping fit was more important now than ever before. Maintaining a heathy weight pre, during and post chemotherapy is important to help protect from breast cancer. Current evidence suggests that breast cancer risk is 30-40% lower amongst women who take regular exercise. The cancer preventative effects of exercise seem to go beyond its impact on weight and may also be linked to lower levels of cancer promoting hormones such as insulin, oestrogen and testosterone.

Two weeks after my diagnosis, I took part in Hellrunner. By this point my life has changed drastically: my long hair had been cut into a bob and I had undergone a lymph node biopsy. When I filled in the application form, never in a million years did I think I would be doing the race with breast cancer. However I felt stronger than ever before on my run, probably because I was determined to do everything in my power to beat the cancer and not let it win. When I completed the race I was exhausted but felt incredible, my body felt so alive and healthy — it was difficult to believe I had cancer. Over the coming months, in between treatments, I continued to run three miles, three to four times a week. It helped keep my mind focused and increased my energy levels, decreasing fatigue, which was particularly important during chemo.

I carried on whenever I could, but it was sometimes hard to do during the intense chemotherapy, so I decided to set myself a challenge to run three miles a day in between treatments during the first half of my chemotherapy treatment. At this stage my chemo was every three weeks and for two out of the three I would just feel tired from the drugs. Setting the challenge was something I did for myself to make me exercise daily. I knew once I decided to do it there was no way I wouldn't complete it. For the next 11 days I went out every day, whatever the weather. There were a few times when I could have so easily not done it because of tiredness and challenging weather conditions (it was the height of winter!), however, I knew how fantastic and proud of myself I would feel having done it and that's what pushed me to see it through to the end. The last day of my challenge was the day before the next round of chemo; completing my final run knowing I had done it filled me with so much happiness and satisfaction. My energy levels had definitely improved and fatigue had decreased. Physically I felt great and, as an added bonus, I had lost a few pounds, ready to take on chemo number 3!

> ***Exercising regularly has many benefits:***
> - Helps prevent weight gain and encourages weight loss;
> - Increases muscular strength and flexibility;
> - Improves self-esteem and confidence;
> - Reduced anxiety and depression;
> - Improves body shape and makes you feel more toned;
> - Reduced risk of heart disease and stroke by 30%;
> - Reduced risk of osteoporosis and arthritis;
> - Reduced risk of diabetes;
> - Better sleeping patterns;
> - Improved balance;
> - Improved fitness;
> - Improved breathing; and
> - Can help your immune system.

Although exercise is important, it is more critical that you don't do too much too soon, and listen to your body, especially during chemotherapy. As I got further into my treatment, my running become less due to the effect treatment was having on my body. However, even though I no longer ran, I still walked regularly and at every opportunity, for example, I would walk instead of driving when picking my little girl up from school, take the steps instead of the escalator when shopping, and park further away from my destination and walk the rest of the way. Sometimes I found walking upstairs to get dressed more tiring than doing any specific exercise.

As well as walking, I did some cardio vascular, strengthening and flexibility exercises alongside my diet plan. This enabled me to make sure that the balance between the energy I took in and energy I burned off was equal, meaning I was more likely to stay the same weight. The best way to lose weight or prevent weight gain is by consuming less energy (calories) and increasing your activity level.

Our metabolic rate is the number of calories we need to function each day — to breathe, digest food, repair cells etc. Chemotherapy can cause a small drop in metabolic rate, which means there is more of a need to watch the calorie intake and try to be more active.

CARDIOVASCULAR EXERCISE

Cardiovascular exercise helps to burn calories and improve fitness and includes activities such as running or walking. It will also help lower the risk of heart disease and some cancers, help lower blood pressure, improve cholesterol levels, burns body fat and is a great healing remedy for stress. Being on your feet is also great for maintaining bone density.

Exercising outdoors has its added benefits, especially in the summer months as exposure to the sun will increase your production of vitamin D. Vitamin D helps the body to absorb calcium, which is essential for good bone health, and also helps the immune, muscle and nervous systems to function properly. Research suggests that women with low levels of the vitamin have a higher risk of breast cancer. Short periods of direct peak exposure, for example, 15 minutes, 3 times of week, can give you more than your recommended daily amount. Another way to get vitamin D is through good food sources.

Foods rich in vitamin D:

- Fortified milk;
- Eggs;
- Cheese;
- Fortified cereal;
- Butter;
- Cream;
- Fish;
- Orange Juice; and
- Oysters

I recommend you do the following warm up before starting cardio vascular, flexibility or strengthening exercises.[3]

---

[3] All exercises are from a booklet I was given along with my B-AHEAD 2 diet — 'Keeping active during chemotherapy.'

WARM-UP
Marching on the spot

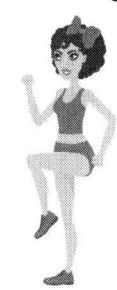

- Stand with your legs shoulder width apart.
- Perform a walking action but lift your knees a little higher and swing your arms up and down in opposition to your legs. (March around the room rather than one spot if you wish.)
- Keep this activity going for 1-2 minutes.

Shoulders

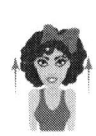

- In sitting or standing position, gently shrug your shoulders as high as you can.
- Relax and repeat 2-4 times.
- Then circle your shoulders first one way and then the other 2-4 times.

Neck Stretches

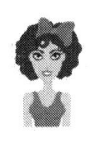

- The neck area is a very delicate area and should not be stretched by circling the head. The following exercises are designed to allow you to stretch the neck area in a safe and controlled manner.
- In sitting or standing position, turn your head as far to one side as is comfortable and until you feel a stretch.
- Hold for 3 seconds.
- Relax and repeat the same on the other side.
- Repeat 2-4 times.

- In sitting or standing position, pull your chin in, keeping your back straight and not tipping your head forwards.
- Hold at the end position and feel the stretch in your neck for 3 seconds.

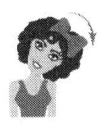

- In sitting or standing position, tilt your head toward one shoulder until you feel the stretch on the opposite side.
- Hold for 3 seconds.
- Relax and repeat to the other side.
- Repeat 2-4 times.

STRENGTHENING EXERCISES

This type of exercise increases muscle mass and improves strength and endurance. More muscle means your metabolic rate is higher so that you burn more calories and improve insulin sensitivity. It's also important for maintaining strong bones and maintaining healthy joints. To increase muscle mass, muscular strength and endurance, aim to do these exercises 2 to 3 times each week. Here are examples of some of the exercises I did regularly.

Single leg lifts

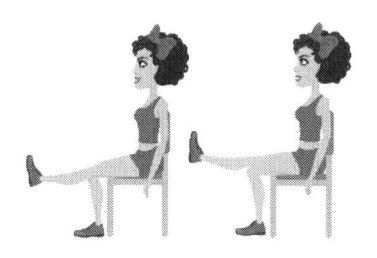

- Sit in a high-backed chair with your back firmly against the back of the chair.
- Straighten one leg then lift it until the thigh comes off the chair.
- Repeat with the other leg.

Step-ups

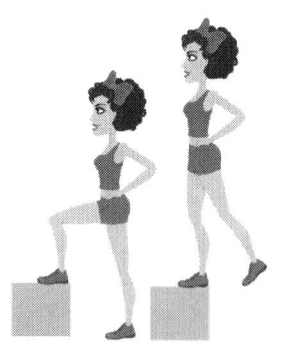

- Find a step or low chair and ensure it is secure and will not move.
- Begin to step up and down on the step. Aim to get your foot flat on the step and lift your weight until the leading leg is straight before stepping down.
- Change which leg leads every so often.
- Keep this going for 1-2 minutes.
- Repeat the exercise.

FLEXIBILITY EXERCISES

Doing these exercises regularly can increase the range of movements in your joints. It is recommended to do the following exercises 2-3 times a week. These exercises would also be in addition to the exercises the physiotherapist would give you just before or after surgery.

The most important thing when exercising is to listen to what your body is telling you. Everybody will respond differently. The best way to gauge your intensity of exercise is to go by how you feel.

Seated hamstring stretch

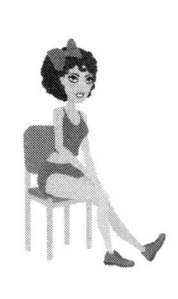

- Sit in an upright position on a chair with your knees bent at a 90 degree angle and both feet resting on the floor.
- Place the heel of your right foot in front of you so that your leg is almost straight, but keep a slight bend in it.
- Very gently lean your upper body forward and place your hands on your left knee.
- Hold the stretch in position for 1-2 minutes. You should feel a gentle stretch up the back of the leg and also in your calf muscle.
- Repeat the exercise using the left leg.

Thigh Stretch

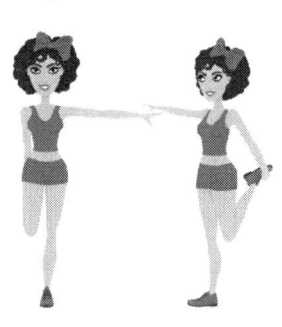

- Stand near a wall (use the wall for support) or lie on one side.
- Bend one knee, bringing the foot towards your bottom, keeping your thighs pressed together. If you can, gently hold on to the arch of your foot with one hand and bring it closer to your bottom until you feel the stretch. If you can't reach your feet, try holding on to your trouser leg instead. You should feel the stretch on the front of your thigh.
- If you can't feel the stretch, then bring your bum closer to your bottom.
- Hold the stretch in this position for 1-2 minutes.
- Repeat this exercise with the other leg.

Triceps stretches

- Either seated or standing, raise your right arm and drop the hand back between the shoulder blades (or behind your head).
- If you can, reach up with your left hand and gently pull your right elbow towards your head. If you can't manage this, lift your left hand up and place it on the back of your right arm and push your right arm back, moving your right hand down your back until you feel a stretch in the back of your right upper arm and shoulder joint.
- Hold the stretch for 1-2 minutes.
- Repeat stretch in this position and then relax.
- Repeat this exercise for the other side.

> For step-by-step instructions, go to ***www.sarahsstory.co.uk*** to receive your free exercise video.

During exercise you should feel slightly warm and be breathing more heavily but should still be able to talk. Making sure you are comfortable with the intensity is vitally important. During the days after chemotherapy you might notice your breathing during exercise feels much heavier, so you may need to reduce the intensity to light or moderate. Use the perceived exertion scale to help you (0-10).

Perceived Exertion Scale

0 = Nothing at all

1 = Very, very light

2 = Very light

3 = Light

4 = Moderate

5 = somewhat hard
(effort is required to maintain a conversation)

6 = Hard

7 = Very hard

8 = Very, very hard

9 = Extremely hard

10 = Absolute maximal effort (no conversation, breathing is hard)

Extracted from 'Keeping active during chemotherapy' — B-AHEAD 2

You may find that you need to break the exercises into small chunks throughout the day; this will enable you to still achieve what you want but without feeling tired. Also remember to take caution on the days you have steroids as they help to reduce the inflammatory response and help reduce the toxic side effects of chemotherapy. Steroids therefore have a placebo effect, giving you false energy.

The great thing about stretching and flexibility exercises are that you can do them inside the house, which is perfect for those days when you don't feel like getting dressed and going outside. Building up your exercise regime needs to be done gradually. It is much more beneficial to take your time and do the exercises properly. That way you make sure you get optimum results.

> *Top tips for exercising safely*
> - Build your exercise programme up slowly to reduce the likelihood of injuries.
> - Don't overexert yourself — signs of overexertion include nausea, sickness, dizziness and chest pain;
> - Always wear loose, comfortable clothing and footwear with a good arch support;
> - Don't eat a big meal before you exercise. Wait at least one hour after eating before exercising;
> - Drink plenty of water before and after exercising;
> - Always stretch on finishing exercise; and
> - Don't exercise if you have a temperature or other signs of an infection.

The best way to get started if you have never done any of these exercises is to start with walking — this is the easiest form of exercise. You should aim to walk at a pace that is comfortable for you but which makes you slightly warm and out of puff. Your walk should be quick and you should still be able to have a conversation.

Aim to walk about 4-5 times a week. It's a good idea to plan your route and to maybe arrange to go with a friend or family member, or even listen to music. I find listening to music helps my mind to relax and stops me from focusing on the exercise and how many miles I've got left until I finish! There are also quite a few walking groups you can go along to.

Twelve months post treatment and I have taken up running again and have recently started a 12-week fitness programme at the local leisure centre. I was informed of the programme by St Luke's hospice in Winsford. The programme is offered to all cancer patients and is absolutely free! I had to get a referral from my GP and, after that, I was put on a short waiting list. To begin, I had my level of fitness assessed by a personal trainer who put a fitness plan in place for me to use over the 12 weeks. I can go to the gym as many times as I like in the twelve weeks and it also includes unlimited swimming sessions.

The 12-week programme has definitely helped my recovery and has pushed me to exercise more frequently. My body has taken some impact from the drugs and trauma, so that if I don't exercise a minimum of three times a week all my muscles tighten up, I get throbbing pains in my arms and legs and everything stiffens.

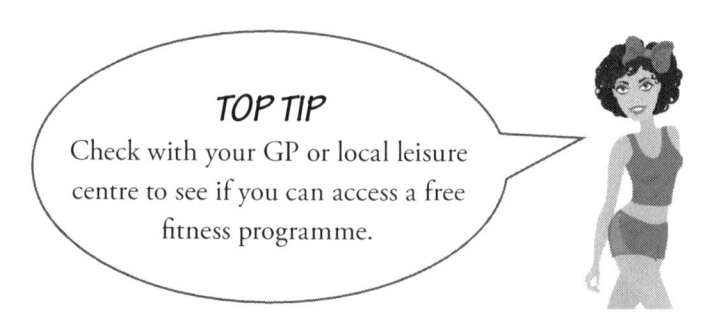

> **TOP TIP**
> Check with your GP or local leisure centre to see if you can access a free fitness programme.

Holistic therapies

I've always been really open-minded when it comes to holistic therapies and homeopathic remedies. After my diagnosis it became apparent that a range of therapies could be used on cancer suffers to help ease anxiety, pain, depression and stress and reduce side effects such as nausea and sickness. There is a wide range of therapies out there to choose from.

Examples of Holistic Therapies

- Acupuncture;
- Aromatherapy
- Art therapy;
- Counselling;
- Dietary supplements;
- Emotional Freedom Technique (EFT);
- Flower remedies;
- Group therapy;
- Healing;
- Herbal remedies;
- Homeopathy;
- Hypnotherapy;
- Massage therapy;
- Mindfulness meditation;
- Music therapy;
- Nutritional therapy;
- Reflexology;
- Reiki;
- Relaxation;
- Self-help groups;
- Shiatsu and acupressure;
- Tai chi and qi gong;
- Therapeutic touch;
- Visualisation; and
- Yoga.

For more information on the above go to www.macmillan.org.uk

---

118 *S Pickles*

So many to choose from so do some research and see if any are right for you. I benefitted from a number of therapies on the list both during and after treatment and will tell you a bit more about them.

Hypnotherapy & EFT

These were therapies I had never experienced before but after meeting a lovely lady called Toni Mackenzie, a counsellor, physiotherapist, NLP practitioner and life coach, I decided to give them a go. Toni and I had only met a couple of times and when she found out about my diagnosis she very kindly offered me a hypnotherapy session to help reduce anxiety, stress and sickness whilst going through chemotherapy.

People with cancer most often use hypnotherapy for sickness or pain as there is some evidence that it helps with these symptoms. It can also help with depression, anxiety and stress. Hypnotherapy is a therapy that uses hypnosis — obvious really. You are in a trance-like state where your body is deeply relaxed but your mind is active.

Toni also showed me a technique called EFT (Emotional Freedom Technique), which is an emotional healing technique that helps to release blockages, allowing you to deal with them. Some examples of these 'blockages' are anxiety, lack of confidence and depression. I used it just before I went for my second MRI Scan after suffering with anxiety and feeling claustrophobic during my first scan. After practising EFT the morning of the second scan, I found it to be a completely different experience and I was totally relaxed.

As well as having hypnotherapy from Toni at the beginning of my diagnosis, I also received hypnosis from a fantastic hypnotherapist called Fraser at St Luke's hospice after my treatment had finished, which helped me deal with the aftermath of diagnosis.

The effects of hypnotherapy were very effective pre- and post- treatment and helped me to deal with anxiety and stress, as well as helping me to deal with what I had been through. I would highly recommend it to help with recovery.

Healing sessions

This came about because I had a friend who specialises in energy healing and natural meditation. He very kindly offered to do some healing sessions on me in the hope that it would have a positive impact on my treatment. I said yes as I was willing to try anything that could be a benefit to my health. I had seven sessions because I had seven tumours.

In the first session, neither of us knew quite what to expect, as this was the first time Chris had worked with somebody going through cancer. I got comfortable, closed my eyes and started to relax as he began the session. The first thing I saw was a pale yellow/green energy; Chris had also seen this moving out of my hands before I told him what I could see. I also saw dark, grey colours, which was energy in the affected area. As Chris removed it my head felt like a dead weight.

Each week Chris would bring something he had a feeling was relevant to the session. For example, one week he brought a pack of angel cards. The card I chose read 'be mindful of the foods you eat' and, two days later I would be starting my B-AHEAD 2 diet!

During the sessions over the next few weeks I saw yellow, green, blue and pink colours, which Chris explained to me was energy. I could also feel when Chris started to 'extract' the tumours, moving through my chest, my head and then out. As each was 'removed', the pressure in my body alleviated. Throughout each session, I had my eyes closed and explained to Chris what I could feel and see.

Halfway through the sessions I had an MRI scan to see if the tumours had shrunk since treatment started and they had. It was impossible to know exactly what positive impact the healing sessions had on my tumours; however, I believe and feel they had helped in some way.

We continued with the last three sessions. Chris began to work on instructing the cells to change their behaviour to help prevent the cancer from returning. Through the session I felt a searing pain; the only way I can describe it is it was as if Chris was pulling something big and heavy out of the top of my head from my chest then, all of a sudden, my head felt as light as a feather. When I relayed this back to Chris he told me he had been working on one of the bigger tumours out of the seven and as he was corkscrewing it out, this was what I could feel.

For anyone who doesn't believe in the power of healing you probably think this is a load of nonsense. However, I say don't knock it until you have tried it! I was fascinated by my experiences throughout the sessions. I strongly believe it has had a positive impact on my final diagnosis; it also helped to calm my mind and body, assisting me to relax at times when I really need it, as well as giving me hope.

Reflexology and Reiki

These treatments were offered by St Luke's Hospice. I had never had reiki before but had heard positive things about the treatment. Reflexology and the Navitas centre was something I was quite familiar with as I have a diploma in it, so I knew it was very effective. However, I didn't quite know the impact it would have on me whilst going through chemotherapy treatment. I was excited to see what the benefits would be as I had heard that complimentary therapies can make you feel stronger and more confident to deal with chemotherapy.

I was allocated a 6-week course — each session consisting of a reiki and reflexology treatment. The therapy room was beautiful and very relaxing. It was enveloped with warm lighting and you could hear soft, gentle relaxation music and smell lavender as you walked in (very different to the ambience at hospital!). My whole body began to unwind and relax as soon as I entered the room, forgetting about everything that I was going through at the time and, for those precious moments of treatment, I felt normal rather than a cancer patient. I removed my wig, making sure I was as comfortable as possible, before getting on the bed as the therapist covered me with a warm, soft blanket — I felt so happy and content.

Mindfulness

One thing I struggled with whilst going through chemotherapy treatment was having time for me and taking the time to relax. I always felt I needed to be doing something whenever I was feeling well enough (especially after spending a few days in bed). Being busy was also my way of coping with what was happening to my body. Generally, as women we always feel it's our job to carry out our daily chores, going above and beyond, taking our role as a mummy and wife very seriously, no matter what gets in our way — 'superwoman' comes to mind! This was exactly what I was still trying to be, even with cancer. In fact, I took my role much more seriously because, if I didn't, I was frightened the 'big C' would get the better of me. (However, sometimes I had to admit defeat and realise it wasn't always possible.) I had to change my mindset and learn 'mindfulness', which is something St Luke's hospice also helped me with during my weekly treatments. By not allowing my body to rest and relax when it needed and by feeling stressed, I would be feeding the cancer. Adjusting my mindset and teaching myself how to switch off my very active mind was not easy. However, I forced myself to do it and found it helped me to slow down my mind and body, helping me to become much more relaxed.

Before each treatment, the therapist would spend 5-10 minutes on some mindfulness techniques to relax me. I would feel like I was sinking through the bed. Each week would be a completely different experience: I would see colours ranging from pinks to yellows and orange. Having the treatments also allowed me to have a chat to the nurse about any concerns and how I was feeling. At the end of the six weeks my body felt completely re-energised and I had mastered mindfulness! I felt so much better physically and mentally and was very appreciative of having had such a wonderful experience and would highly recommend it.

(Web links to all businesses and hospice that are mentioned within the holistic section can be found at the back of the book.)

> **TOP TIP**
> Using a variety of holistic therapies, including hypnotherapy and healing, all helped to reduce my fear and anxiety, increased my sense of wellbeing and made the side effects such as sickness much easier to manage. Why not see what works for you?

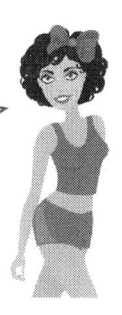

Family and friends

Family and friends play an important role in our lives. They can influence how we are feeling by saying the 'right' or 'wrong' things, make us laugh, pick us off the floor when we're feeling really low, comfort us with open arms and tell us everything is going to be OK. They can be a shoulder to cry on and sometimes the best thing they can do is to tell us to stop feeling sorry for ourselves, to get a grip, pull up our big girl knickers and just get on with it.

> My husband and my daughter meant that it wasn't an option for me not to survive. And now I feel much stronger and I can start living again

After been diagnosed with breast cancer, I really started to understand the true importance of family and friends and the impact their support, love and care had on me whilst going through treatment, especially Dave and Lillie, who both became my strength. (I still can't believe Lillie was only four-years-old when I was diagnosed and how brave she was.) As a family you will go through so much together, as well as individually. It's a difficult time for everybody, but especially you. Sometimes it can become frustrating because you don't always feel you can express yourself openly because nobody will understand, however it is better to talk openly about how you are feeling.

No matter how much you try to communicate with your friends and family, sometimes it feels as if no one else fully understands what you are going through. However, it could also be the case for your loved ones. They may feel powerless, upset, confused and angry, and yet they are trying to keep a brave face for you. Because of this, I asked my lovely husband, Dave, to write down his side of the story. This is what he had to say…

Dave's story

I looked at Sarah and smiled lovingly — what a great night's sleep! It was a beautiful day with the sun shining and a slight breeze — autumn was definitely in the air. We woke up and got ready for Sarah's appointment at hospital to find out the results of her mammogram. We were a bit nervous but very much full of excitement for our future plans; as work was going well for both of us, we felt settled, my fitness training was great and our daughter, Lillie, was thriving and loving life.

As we got into the car I started to feel that this could be serious and we may come back to our home changed forever. I didn't believe it, but my life experiences from being in the outdoors and being on deployments with the military had taught me you should 'never say never'. Being a born optimist, preparing for a 'What-if' was very much a learned skill.

Walking through the hospital and into the waiting room I went into 'preparation and protection mode' to preserve my wellbeing just in case things didn't go well. Sarah and I sat down and I remember trying to keep her mind occupied with a National Geographic magazine, but I felt that Sarah was also thinking about the 'What-if' too. Sarah was called in to the consultation room, so we stood and made our way through and sat down as the door closed behind us. Shortly after, a nurse appeared and asked Sarah if she had had her operation yet! I distinctly remember thinking, 'What on earth was that all about?' The consultant came in, along with another nurse who was dressed differently. Generally being third-party aware, I clocked her name badge above it. It said 'Macmillan nurse'. I braced myself as Sarah and I held hands so tightly that we had cut off the blood supply long ago. The fog came down and blood seemed to instantly drain from my body — a brilliant body blow ripped out my heart and stole some of its innocence forever.

The following hour was gruelling and gnarly. I felt incredibly protective over Sarah and wanted to take all her pain, upset and suffering away and carry it myself. There is simply nothing worse than seeing another human being who you selflessly love being smashed to bits as though in a car crash.

I held Sarah so tight, with her head to my chest, while she sobbed her heart out and I could feel a whole host of emotions coming from her, including anger and complete helplessness.

We drove home after discussing what the general treatment plan was for Sarah. Fortunately, at the time I had Sarah on my private health insurance so we had more treatment options than usually available on the NHS.

Generally speaking I can't remember much more of that day as I think my learnt preservation switch had flicked and I went into military mode, which was reactive rather than consciously engaged. It was a logical day and I tried very hard to supress my hurt because I knew instantly that this would be an endurance event of epic proportions.

As Sarah and I had been trying for a second child, we went through IVF before Sarah then went onto chemotherapy and then on to having surgery. Nineteen days later I was to run the Chester Marathon with two friends, Pete Leak and Amy Hamblin. Sarah wanted me to still run as we had been training hard. I also felt that in times of great challenge, it isn't what happens, it's how we deal with it. So the three of us ran and had a special shared experience where everything for me was now super-charged. At times it was emotionally very difficult as Sarah's diagnosis of breast cancer kept pushing its way into the forefront of my mind. Sarah and my mum kept appearing at various spectator points, which was brilliant, and when I saw them at the finish line, I nearly fell apart. Hugging Sarah brought back feelings and memories of when I saw her and held her after coming back from a military deployment a few years before — it was quite simply a very pure, happy and deeply connected moment.

Three weeks later I was due to lead a group of people up Kilimanjaro. Again, Sarah wanted me to go because others were depending on me. I have now been up Kilimanjaro 48 times and I can quite honestly say that that trip was the toughest I have ever experienced. I absolutely hated being away from Sarah and it felt so wrong. Luckily, there were some wonderful people on the trip, including close friends, who showed real compassion and support for me and my situation.

The Kilimanjaro trip was a success but now I was 100% focused on getting back to Sarah, who was due to have her eggs harvested after the IVF preparation phase. The preparation phase itself was gruelling, as anyone could tell you who has been through IVF. Injecting a needle into your loved-one's tummy is never a 'turn-on' for either person.

Now, regards to my 'personal donation' to the IVF process, it was full of laughs and 'interesting' moments, but for the purpose of this story I will fast forward to me landing at London Heathrow airport on my return from Kilimanjaro. I immediately caught a bus to Reading, picked up my car and drove to St. Mary's hospital in Manchester as fast as I could (but keeping to the speed limit of course). The aim was to get to Sarah, who was having her eggs harvested in time for my arrival if possible. Even though I had donated my sperm already and it seemed to be top quality rated (grrr...manly), it was frozen and, ideally they wanted a 'fresh donation.'

Upon my arrival, I jumped out of the car and ran up the flights of stairs to *see Sarah just coming round as she recovered from the operation. As I gave her a broad smile, massive hug and a kiss I gradually became aware there was someone else standing by the bed. (Remember the 'third-party awareness?) I turned slowly to see the senior staff nurse observing me from head to toe (I was still wearing my walking gear with dust on my boots). "Are you Mr David Pickles?" she asked. Once my identity was verified she asked me to go down to the appropriate department and provide a fresh donation of sperm. This request was asserted in front of other people on the ward and was quite a welcome back to the UK! I seem to remember that even the cleaner looked at me with a smile and a snigger, along with the patients, doctors and nurses, who were all within earshot.*

So I went to the 'appropriate department' as quickly as I could and assumed the appropriate stance and focus. All I will say is that even though we had a very slim chance to no chance at all of having any success with IVF, we now have two fertilised embryos waiting to be used. It seems that there was a reason for me to go up Kilimanjaro as my three-second hard work provided a fresh donation that was good quality stuff!

The days, weeks and months rolled on at a painfully slow and deeply upsetting rate. They were the darkest days I have ever experienced in my life and it was the hardest time I have ever had to endure. I became a carer for Sarah, a mother and father to Lillie, all at the same time as having to hold my job down, keep the house in order and make sure Lillie was affected by this ordeal as little as possible. Because of the stress, worry and upset, my wellbeing was smashed and eventually started to exploit weaknesses in my body. I had a back relapse (a lower herniated disc which is an on-going situation), which added physical pain to the mental and emotional pain. I had to work so hard in keeping things together and it certainly took its toll. From a male perspective I am happy to express my emotions and talk about problems but this was all very different. Nothing prepared me for what was needed of me and I don't feel anything can. We really get to know ourselves when faced with remote and austere environments and challenges and this environment was so alien to me. I discovered that I wasn't as strong as I hoped I was and also that it's OK to show cracks, but to not let them turn into chasms. I found that the most important resource is to engage your moral compass and to exact core values such as courage and compassion, as well as to focus on and protect the innocents in the situation 100% of the time, which in this case were Sarah and Lillie.

Sarah and I, over the years, have worked hard to compromise with each other and make room for each other to be who we are and to grow. We have supported each other, even when it may not have been the course of action we wanted to take, but to fundamentally love each other selflessly. All this came into the forefront and, as a result, we hung on as a family and, no matter what we believed, we would come out of the other end better, stronger, healthier and happier. After all, never giving up is the only option.

It's very difficult to know everything will be OK. When in really tough and critical situations, my training had taught me to keep moving forward; when it comes to beating cancer there is no other choice but to fully engage hope, faith and blind belief that everything will be good again. Faith and hope are very personal things, but I would strongly suggest you take a step back and think about what your core values of faith and hope are, because you never know when you will need them most, either for yourself or for others.

I have always believed and felt that by helping others it will bring true happiness and balance. These things were critical to my survival as a carer to Sarah and as Daddy to Lillie.

It is important to keep the basics going, which are good nutrition, correct hydration, the right amount of sleep and regular exercise. Fresh air will ease the stress away, even if it's only temporary.

Everyone going through cancer with a loved one will feel slightly different compared to someone else's experience, even if on paper they are going through the same situation. If you are lucky enough to have a great family support network around you that can help take the pressure off then perfect, but for anyone who doesn't have that, you need to try and find ways of decompressing and recharging, even with seemingly insignificant things. I love gardening and being in the outdoors, so when I got a chance I would go out into the garden and potter around. The times I could do this were few and far between but it really did help. Our journey as a family was during the winter months, so this became another compounding issue and another layer of test.

One thing I would absolutely advise against is not taking charge of the situation. This is essential for survival reasons and will help carry you forward over the whole gnarly experience of surviving cancer as a family. Research the cancer your loved one has and find alternative therapies. Conventional medicine is good but unconventional treatments, when mixed with conventional, is outstanding. There are so many non-evasive treatments out there that really do work and do not be afraid to use them. The one question I always asked the medical professional was, "Will it be a detriment to Sarah's health or potentially trigger cancer to come back again?" Do not take the *word of one person as gold and make sure you get three opinions at least. To beat a bad situation, it often pays to be bold in thought as well as heart. I annoyed so many medical professionals by constantly asking them questions and discussing other things I had found out. I have a deep respect for the medical profession and the NHS, as both the individuals and this wonderful institution do an incredible job. However, please remember that no one cares as much as you do about your loved one and it is your responsibility to do everything possible because you only get one chance at smashing cancer into touch. It is a despicable disease and I believe lifestyle has a hand to play in it, so look for sustainable options which work well. Life is the most precious of gifts and should be cherished and loved. There is so much more to say and so much more detail to our journey as a family and mine as a carer but ultimately never ever give up and keep moving forward. When everything goes dark, just go as far as you can and then go a little further — keep breathing, keep living, keep hope, keep faith.*

The following quote by Sir Winston Churchill defines how important courage is and what an incredible tool it is in beating anything:

"Success isn't final, failure isn't fatal: it's the courage to continue that really counts."

Family and friends may want to help but find it difficult to understand what you're going through and may be worried they may say or do the wrong thing. Communicating with each other is really important, even though sometimes you don't feel like it. This will make it much easier for the people around you to respond to your needs. Don't be afraid to take advantage of any help offered from friends and family or be scared to ask for help.

How to respond to "What can I do for you?"

- Cooking;
- Cleaning;
- Listening;
- Washing/ironing;
- Shopping;
- Picking up your prescriptions;
- Chauffeur you to hospital appointments;
- Chemotherapy buddy;
- Washing and blow drying your wig; and
- Filing and Polishing your nails.

Something I found difficult was people walking in the opposite direction when they saw me, but I soon realised it wasn't because they didn't like me anymore, they just didn't know what to say — so try not to be offended. It's not intentional; everybody reacts very differently and in ways you least expect.

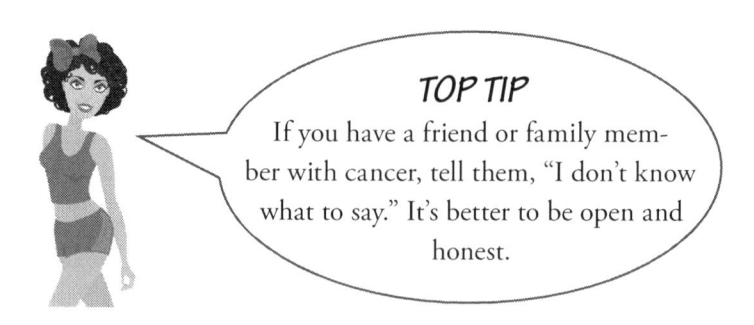

> **TOP TIP**
> If you have a friend or family member with cancer, tell them, "I don't know what to say." It's better to be open and honest.

This is my own quote and what I lived by each day:

> *'When you're feeling vulnerable, look at the people you love and turn your vulnerability into strength to enable you to move forward, keep focused, be determined and to Never Give Up.'*
> Sarah Pickles

When I was diagnosed, I wanted to do everything I could to give me the best chance of beating breast cancer. I believe that watching my diet, exercise and being open-minded to holistic therapies all played a part in my recovery. Also, being open, honest and accepting help from friends and family when it was offered was crucial to me every step of the way.

The other factor that gave me strength to deal with everything on this difficult journey and to mentally give myself the best chance was to look good whenever I could. I will tell you a bit more about that in my next chapter…step into my beauty salon!

CHAPTER NINE

Looking Good, Feeling Great

Throughout my journey, I never underestimated the importance of looking good to help me feel good. A slash of lipstick and a pretty dress gave me an instant boost and helped me feel like I could take on the world.

However, cancer and chemotherapy can ravage your body, making you feel terrible and look drained, so the last thing you want to do is get dolled up and go out. But I say give it a go. Even if you are feeling awful, even if you just want to hide away from the world — don't! Get dressed up, slap on some lipstick and leave the house. You will feel better for it.

Of course, there will be days when you really can't budge — fair enough. Just make sure you take care of yourself. In this chapter I will give you some hints and tips of how to look after your skin and how I adapted my beauty regime to keep looking good during chemotherapy treatment.

'No matter how you feel, get up, dress up, show up and never give up'
Anon

I knew that chemotherapy, as well as making my hair fall out, was also going to change the appearance of my body and the condition of my skin and nails. This meant my finger and toenails could develop ridges and become brittle and could even fall off. Also, the steroids could make my skin become sensitive, red and prone to spots.

After my second chemotherapy I noticed my skin become very pale, sometimes red, more sensitive to light, dry and dehydrated.

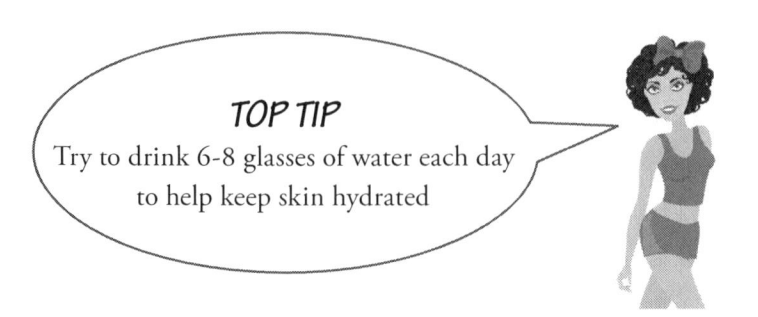

> **TOP TIP**
> Try to drink 6-8 glasses of water each day to help keep skin hydrated

How to look after dry skin

- Use gentle, fragrance-free soaps that will help prevent your skin from drying out more (bathing in 'Oilatum' helps to moisturise, condition and protect the skin);
- Use a facial cleanser that won't strip the moisture out of your skin;
- Clean your body with lukewarm water as hot water dries out the skin;
- Remove cleanser with damp cotton wool;
- Don't exfoliate your skin when it is dry as it will dehydrate even more;
- If using a toner, make sure it doesn't contain alcohol as this will dry the skin further; and
- Using a moisturiser daily can help reduce dry skin — look out for moisturisers with ceramides, cholesterol, glycerine, hyaluronic acid.

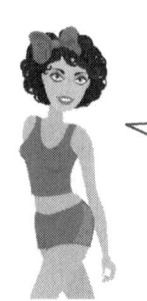

> **TOP TIP**
> Mixing a couple of drops of vitamin E oil in with your moisturiser will help reduce dryness, fine lines and wrinkles.

As I've said before, it is so important to get out in the fresh air and sunlight. It all helps to make you feel better and helps you to produce that all-important vitamin D. However, you need to be aware that your skin may be even more sensitive to the sun and you need to make sure you use a sunscreen with a high SPF (SPF 30+), and also that you remember to put it everywhere — including your scalp and neck. I made the mistake of forgetting to do just that and got burnt whilst camping in Wales because I under-estimated the weather. It was sunny but a bit overcast with a cool wind so I didn't think I would burn like I did; however, I did and this resulted in me having lots of pain in my arm where I had the lymph nodes removed. For at least a week I experienced a deep throbbing pain, which meant I had to take painkillers to ease the discomfort. I can't stress the importance enough of applying sunscreen whenever the sun is out and continuing with this for the rest of your life.

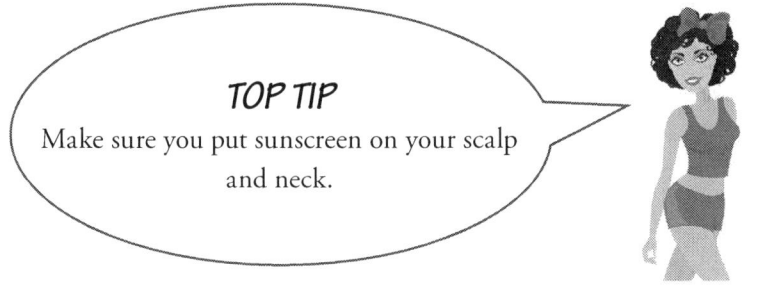

TOP TIP

Make sure you put sunscreen on your scalp and neck.

More tips on how to look after you skin

- Use petroleum jelly or lip balm to keep lips moist and to stop them becoming sore and dry — I would highly recommend using a lip conditioner that contains aloe vera and jojoba;
- Protect yourself from the sun with Factor SP 50 and a minimum of SP 30; and
- Wear a hat or scarf when it's sunny.

It made me realise that looking after my skin was more important than ever before. There are times when looking good on the outside becomes important to allow you to feel and look beautiful as well as giving you confidence — going through breast cancer was definitely one of those times! The only thing I was sure of when I got my diagnosis was that I would always look my best whenever I attended any hospital appointments and especially on chemo days. (There was absolutely no way chemo was going to come between me and my make-up!)

I had no idea at the beginning of my diagnosis the effects chemo would have on my physical appearance but soon it all became apparent. Make–up became my mask whenever I was feeling vulnerable and needed something to hide behind. As the time went on I noticed changes to my skin tone and texture. This meant having to make changes to my make-up application, especially my foundation. Wearing foundation emphasised the dryness of my skin, making my face look more aged. I stopped wearing foundation and changed over to a bb crème, which is a tinted moisturiser that had an SPF 20 and contained Aloe Vera, which was great as it helped nourish my skin.

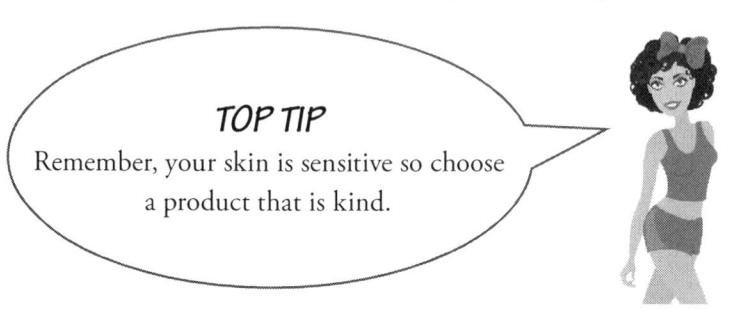

TOP TIP
Remember, your skin is sensitive so choose a product that is kind.

Hints when using foundation

- Your skin will probably change during treatment and may become a different tone. Change the shade of your foundation to match;
- Test foundation on your jawline to help you choose the correct shade for your skin tone. (Leave it for a few minutes to let it absorb into the skin before you make the decision.);
- Choose a liquid foundation if your skin is dry and a cream to powder if your skin is oily;
- If you don't wear a lot of make-up you can use a tinted moisturiser to help even out your skin tone (Choose one that has and SPF in it as this will help to protect your skin too!); and
- If your skin is red, use a green-tinted primer. (To avoid a green face and looking like Shrek, use small amounts and pat gently into the skin.)

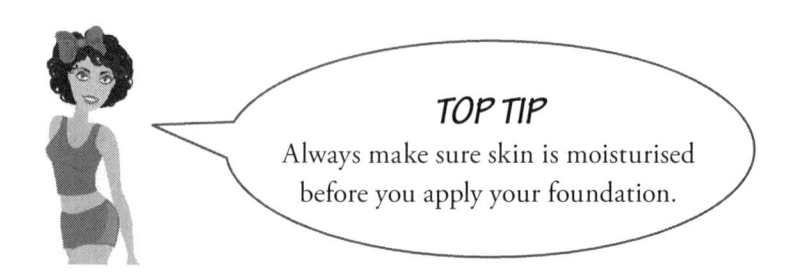

TOP TIP
Always make sure skin is moisturised before you apply your foundation.

As time went on, some days I found that just wearing a bit of bronzer with some blush was enough to give me a healthy glow and helped me to feel better.

> ***Bronzer and blusher tips***
> - When applying bronzer, apply gradually to cheeks, chin and forehead;
> - Use a larger brush to apply more evenly; and
> - When applying blusher, use a smaller brush and apply to the apples of the cheeks.

> **TOP TIP**
> Smiling helps to enhance the cheekbones, making it easy to know exactly where to apply the blusher.

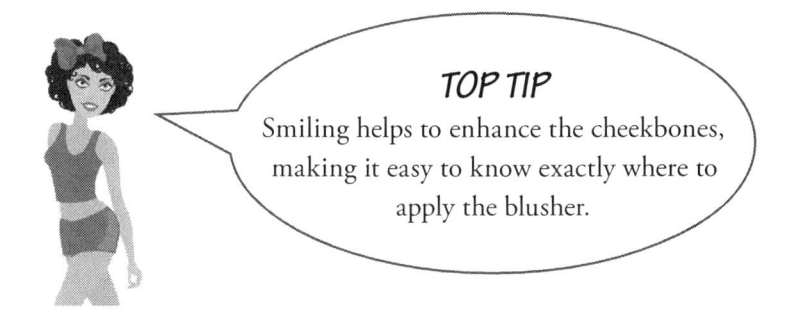

Before I was diagnosed, being a nail technician and passionate about nails, I always wore acrylic nails. It was really difficult having to accept that for the next few months I could no longer wear artificial nails. It took me a few weeks to get used to being without my long nails but I would never have worn false nails through chemotherapy due to the damage they cause to natural nails and the chemicals in the products used. I eventually accepted that I would just have to settle for wearing nail polish for the next few months

My Macmillan nurse advised me to wear a dark nail varnish due to the effects chemotherapy can have on your nails, making them become brittle and flaky, sometimes even changing in shape and colour or becoming sore, resulting in them falling off.

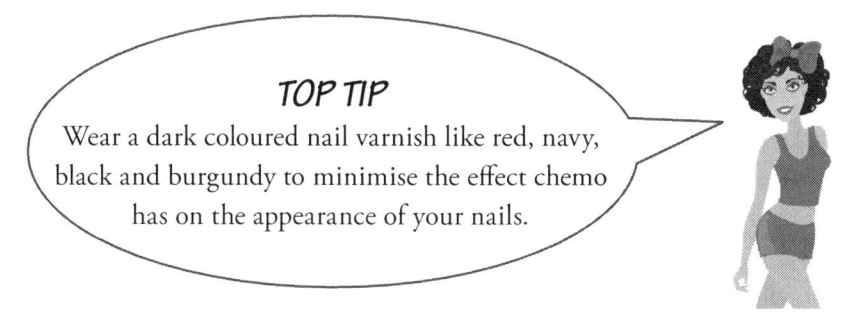

> **TOP TIP**
> Wear a dark coloured nail varnish like red, navy, black and burgundy to minimise the effect chemo has on the appearance of your nails.

The Shock Factor

How to protect your nails during treatment

- Wear a base coat to prevent nails from going yellow and a top coat to seal the polish and prevent chipping;
- Do not cut the cuticles in case you cut the skin;
- File nails using an emery board, filing in one direction across the nail and not by using a sawing action. This will help prevent further damage to your nails;
- Wear gloves when doing household chores e.g. washing the dishes and gardening (too much exposure to water can lead to fungal infection in the nail bed);
- Rubbing an oil or cream with vitamin E into your nails and cuticles helps to prevent dryness, splitting and flaking; and
- Use a hand and foot moisturiser which contains vitamin E.

TOP TIP

Smother your feet and hands in a deep conditioning moisturiser (as natural as possible) and sleep in a pair of socks and gloves. The heat will open up the pores, allowing the cream to penetrate through to the underneath layer of skin (dermis).

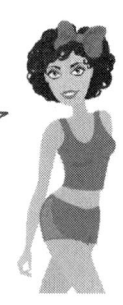

There were a few products I used pre, during and post chemotherapy treatment and also after surgery which definitely improved the condition of my skin and body because of their ingredients.

Propolis Cream — kept my skin well moisturised and reduced dryness.

100% inner leaf Aloe Vera — reduced redness and soothed areas that were sore, tender and itchy (including my scalp when my hair fell out), especially after surgery. It also seemed to help to reduce my scarring.

Aloe Vera lip conditioner — kept my lips super soft and prevented them from going dry and sore.

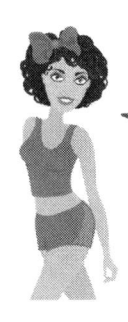

> **TOP TIP**
> Store aloe vera gelly in the fridge and use as a cooling facemask to reduce redness and puffiness around eyes. Leave on the skin for 10 minutes then remove with warm water.

Moisturising serum — used this in my daily facial routine to keep my skin moisturised and on my scalp to condition and prevent it from going dry. A 2-in-1 serum and moisturiser, which not only contains Aloe Vera but also white tea extract, is best, as it has antioxidant and anti-aging properties that help in maintaining good health and healthy skin. It also protects skin from the harmful effects of UV light.

The unique ingredient in each of the above products is Aloe Vera (100% inner leaf), which has a number of beneficial properties.

100% inner leaf Aloe Vera may contribute to the following:

- Anti-Viral
- Anti-Itch
- Anti-fever
- Anti-Fungal
- Anti-Bacterial

During treatment your skin becomes very sensitive and products you have used before may cause irritation as they could contain chemicals that are too harsh for the skin. It is very important that you can find a product that is free of any nasties (harsh chemicals) and gentle on the body. There will be lots of natural and naturally inspired products out there; find the ones that are right for you. I can only relate to my experiences and the benefits I had from using products that contain the natural substances I've listed. I hope that sharing them here will also help you.

If you would like more information about the products, please visit *www.sarahsstory.co.uk*

I remember turning up to my first chemo feeling fabulous. I was rocking my latest hairstyle (a bob), my favourite pair of FatFace flared jeans and a pale pink jumper and a pair of heels. I felt gorgeous and ready to take on the world, completely unaware that a few hours later I would be in my pyjamas, in bed, feeling and looking absolutely awful. Although that happened, it didn't put me off turning up to my next chemo two weeks later all dressed up again, this time in a vintage leopard print skater dress that I had bought a few weeks before from a beautiful vintage boutique called Didi's (I've put website address at the bottom of this page just in case you want to treat yourself!) with a pair of ankle boots with a 4-inch heel and rocking my new red wig. Even though this time I knew that in a few hours I was probably going to be in exactly the same situation as I was two weeks previously, it was important for me to feel good just for those couple of hours whilst having treatment. Next time you have chemo, try it and go glam! You will feel like you can take on the world!

> *I believe a woman is at her most beautiful when she is confident, empowered and strong.*

Over the weeks there was not one chemo session when I didn't dress for the occasion. Although chemo was not a lunch date and made me feel like crap continuously, I didn't want the way I felt inside to make the decision on how I dressed. (If that were the case, I probably would have worn a zombie costume to signify how I was really feeling.)

So, for each treatment or medical appointment (and, quite often, just when leaving the house), I made sure I looked my best, wearing make-up, having my nails painted and wearing a pair of heels! I also made sure that one or two items of clothing I had on were bold and colourful, mostly red and pink. Pink is my favourite colour; it fills me with so much happiness. Red makes me feel strong, confident and in control. Red was a colour I always wore whenever I had an important business meeting before I was diagnosed, whenever I needed to seal the deal. However, it wasn't long before red became my secret weapon throughout treatment — my red lipstick being the most powerful, protecting me from bad news whenever I felt fragile and vulnerable and never leaving my handbag because I never knew when I was going to need it.

> *One of my 'go-to' websites for a new dress to make me look and feel fabulous was Didi's Boutique, who specialise in vintage reproduction and rockabilly* **www.lovedidis.co.uk**

Of course there were times throughout treatment, especially after chemo, when I didn't always have the energy to get dressed or even brush my teeth, never mind putting on make–up. However, this definitely made me feel worse mentally. These were the days I struggled emotionally, seeing myself without make-up because of how ill I looked — completely unrecognisable — not knowing the person staring back at me in the mirror. Chemo had certainly succeeded in changing the condition and appearance of my skin and body. However, I knew this was the way I had to look at the times when I was feeling most unwell.

Whenever my energy levels increased, even if I wasn't leaving the house, I would make the effort to get myself dressed in some casual clothes, put on some mascara (up until I lost my eyelashes, then it was false lashes), and a bit of bronzer and blusher. Applying make–up was more about how it affected my mindset as opposed to vanity. Although physically I was still feeling terrible, mentally I felt better and back in control.

Over the months, my make–up application took more time and effort as I had to pencil in my eyebrows and glue on my eyelashes. This was something I really had to adjust to, as I didn't wear false eyelashes that often before I lost my own because they made my eyes look really small.

Losing your eyelashes and eyebrows is upsetting and really changes your identity but always remember they will grow back and probably better that before.

If your eyelashes do fall out or become thinner, here are a couple of things you can try:
- Applying false eyelashes.
- Using a soft eyeliner pencil and smudger to define your eyes and create the illusion of eyelashes.

*For step-by-step instructions go to **www.sarahsstory.co.uk** to receive your free tutorial.*

As well as losing my eyelashes, I also lost my eyebrows, which meant I had to start pencilling them in. At first I couldn't get used to my drawn-on eyebrows and rocked the 'no eyebrow' look for a while, but then I realised I needed to get used to drawing them on because I looked weird without them! There are two ways you can draw on your eyebrows:
- Using an eyebrow pencil; and
- Applying eyeshadow using a make-up brush.

The Shock Factor

Make sure you use a colour slightly lighter than your hair colour; this makes them look more natural. If you are struggling with the shape, you can buy eyebrow stencils and experiment with different outlines.

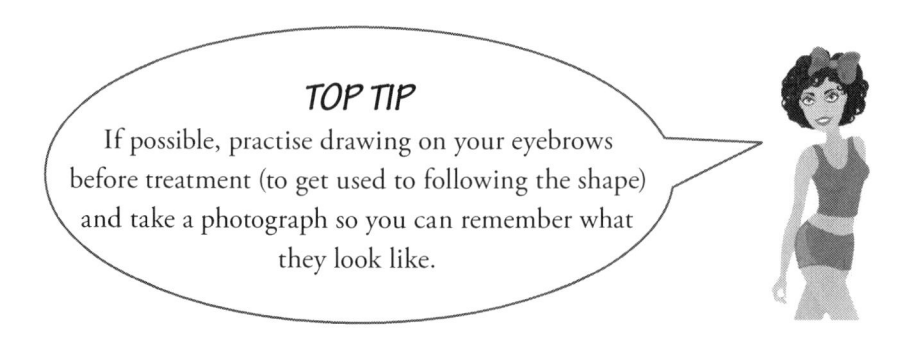

TOP TIP
If possible, practise drawing on your eyebrows before treatment (to get used to following the shape) and take a photograph so you can remember what they look like.

*For step-by-step instructions go to **www.sarahsstory.co.uk** to receive your free tutorial.*

It wasn't long before I adjusted to my new eyebrows and had lots of fun drawing them on and trying out new shapes — this was a positive to losing all my hair, including facial hair, it allowed me to experiment with different styles.

As time went on I began to rely on my make-up more and more. It gave me something to hide behind, making me feel safe, happy and human, not like somebody who had cancer.

Although I liked to wear make-up and to dress up I also really enjoyed taking it all off when I got back to the safety of my home. As I removed my pretty dresses, took off my heels, then filled the cotton wool pad with cleanser and began to remove my make-up bit by bit, it was like wiping a dusty mirror (actually, most days it was more like a smeared window, because I had more and more make-up on which smudged across my face). I began to see this sick person peeking through. It filled me with so much unhappiness seeing myself looking so bare and feeling so empty. However I had to remember that I was alive and kicking cancer's butt. I knew that eventually I would return back to my normal self, but for now I had to accept this was who I was. . .

CHAPTER TEN

Planning Ahead

Before my diagnosis, Dave and I had been trying for a second child. All things considered, it was lucky we had been unsuccessful, as this would have caused a lot of complications. Amongst all the fear and confusion of being told I had cancer was the pain of thinking that the option of having any more children could now be closed to me.

We decided to undergo 'in vitro fertilisation' (IVF) before I started chemotherapy (which can affect your fertility) so that, if everything else went according to plan, we could possibly try again in the future.

It was just three weeks after diagnosis and my day was booked up with hospital appointments. My first appointment was at the doctor's surgery for my flu jab and then Dave and I had an appointment at the IVF clinic at St Mary's Hospital in Manchester; this was our first visit to start discussing the process of IVF.

We arrived at St Mary's in good time, which allowed us to spend some quality time together catching up and absorbing recent events. We hadn't had much time to do this since my diagnosis. It was a bit like having a date night but at the fertility clinic! While we were waiting we were both taking in what was going on around us, watching couples come and go, wondering what their circumstances were and whether their outcome had been a positive one.

I know a few people who had to go through the IVF process, some of whom have had positive results when they have conceived through IVF but then also naturally 12 months later — others have not been so successful. At that point I wasn't the least bit concerned that IVF wouldn't work for us as we had conceived naturally and very easily with our little girl, Lillie. In fact, she was actually conceived whilst I was taking the contraceptive pill!

The doctor explained the IVF process and why it is recommended for women who have been diagnosed with breast cancer and will be having chemotherapy. IVF is a process by which eggs are removed from your ovaries and mixed with sperm in a laboratory culture dish. Fertilisation takes place in this dish, 'in vitro', which literally means 'in glass'. Women who have chemotherapy treatment can become infertile afterwards but also your ovaries age by five years which can then make it harder to conceive. I never thought, at 32 years of age, I would be having IVF or even battling with breast cancer — it was definitely not a part of my lifelong plan.

After we had finished chatting with the doctor I had to give blood and then go for a scan so they could have a look at my ovaries and see how many eggs I had. While we were waiting, another nurse was explaining where I needed to go for my scan. I heard my number being called and, before I could even get out my chair, a loud, booming voice rolled down the corridor, repeating my number. I felt quite scared of this approaching 'sergeant major'. Expecting a rather large, angry nurse, I was surprised when a petite and unassuming lady with a voice that comically sounded like 'Darth Vader' from 'Star Wars' appeared. I looked over at Dave to gauge his facial expression, he looked as shocked and scared by the whole experience as I was! This amused me so much that I had no control as tears of laughter started to roll down my face.

Monday, 13th October 2014

I can't believe we had such a laugh at the IVF clinic! This sergeant major of a nurse had scared Dave and I to death with her booming voice and, just when I started to control my laughter (it must have been nerves), she picked up a file and called out the name on the front – which wasn't even mine!

With a confused look on her face, she asked me to repeat my name. All I could think of was what her blood testing skills were going to be like, if she can't even get my name right?

While she was searching for the correct file I took in the ambience of the room; I could hear the sound of a running tap and was very confused as to why it was constantly running and hadn't been turned off? Surely she could hear the noise? How was it not bothering her? I had only been in there for ten minutes and it was driving me crazy! All I could think of was the amount of water being wasted; even the classical music playing in the background couldn't drown out the sound. I looked out of the window to see bars on the panes of glass and metal spikes on the windowsill. Was this was to stop the patients from escaping? It was like being in a scene from 'Hostel' and soon I would be having my limbs cut off one by one! Well, your imagination does go wild in times of stress!

Eventually the nurse found my file and the blood-taking could commence. My body stiffened and I took a deep breath, worried about whether the needle was going to go in gently. I needn't have worried as she got the needle in first time!

Blood taken, we headed off to the new building for my scan, giggling all the way like school children. We arrived at the maternity department and waited to be called through for the ultrasound. It felt very strange being in this part of the hospital knowing that I wasn't pregnant. While we were waiting we were chatting about how odd it felt to know that we were now about to embark on another journey — IVF — a completely different journey to the one we were already on as this was going to be a happy and exciting one with no horrible barriers to get in our way. We both thought the next time we would be having an internal ultrasound scan would be when I was pregnant with our second child. How different life had become in just three short weeks.

There were so many couples coming and going, some who were in the early stages of pregnancy, some who looked like they were about to give birth any moment and some who were in a similar situation to me but without the complication of cancer!

We were eventually called through to have the scan. The nurse greeted us and then asked me to get undressed and climb onto the bed. Everything was very familiar from when we had Lillie, only this time there wasn't as much excitement because we knew we weren't going to be seeing our baby on the screen. This scan was going to check my egg count in each of my ovaries.

After about 10 minutes of being poked and prodded the scan was finished. The nurse didn't really give too much away and wrote down the results of what she had found on a form. On the way back over the old building of St Mary's we had a sneak peak at what the nurse had written down and, from an unprofessional point of view, everything looked OK. I had eggs in each ovary so everything was fine…or so we thought.

Dr Fitzgerald explained what the scan had found; it was not what we had expected to hear. The scan had shown that my right ovary had no eggs and in my left ovary I only had four eggs, which for someone of my age was extremely low — a women of my age should have about 24 eggs.

He explained that this can be common in a BRCA carrier. At this point I had no idea if I was a BRCA carrier or not as I still hadn't had the test, however it was looking more and more likely that I was. (Little did I know at that time that this was not the case.) This changed everything; the percentage of the IVF working now was very small. I couldn't believe what we were hearing. Dave and I were both on an emotional and physical rollercoaster that neither of us could control. I felt like I had just had another kick to the stomach; not only was I having to come terms with the fact that I had breast cancer, I was now having to accept that I may never be able to have another child and was actually very lucky to have conceived Lillie.

The decision was now in our hands as to whether we still wanted to go ahead with IVF knowing there was only a 1% chance of them retrieving any eggs. But this also meant that, with the extra tests, it would delay chemotherapy by two weeks. We both knew we still wanted to go ahead with IVF, even with the 1% chance. However we needed to find out whether taking the risk and postponing chemotherapy treatment was going to be a detriment to my health and, if this was the case, then we both knew that IVF was not an option as my health was much more important and absolute number one priority. We already have a beautiful daughter and if she is all we are supposed to have then that is how it is meant to be.

A few days later we were given the good news that we could go ahead with IVF as a two-week delay on chemo would not be a major problem. The wheels were put in motion and the following week we were back at St Mary's signing all the consent forms. There was a lot of paperwork and many questions that made both Dave and I feel very uncomfortable — it felt like confession! After the forms were completed we sat back until the nurse called me through. While we were waiting, Dave and I sat there having a giggle about the fact that at some point Dave was going to have do the do — much to his dismay!

We were taken into a small room at the end of the hallway. Then there was another explanation — this time to describe the procedure over the next two weeks. All IVF treatments have to begin with a course of hormone therapy to stimulate the development of several follicles in the ovary. These are collected as eggs, which are then fertilised in a test-tube ('in vitro') to create a number of embryos. After between two and five days in an incubator, one or two of these embryos are transferred through the vagina to the uterus, where implantation occurs and pregnancy begins. However, in IVF as in natural conception, not every embryo implants to become a pregnancy, which is why surplus embryos are frozen — so that you can try again if the first one fails. However, in my situation I had no follicles in one ovary and only three in the other; this was why the course of treatment only stood a 1% chance.

The first step was for me to be given a drug to suppress my natural cycle, which I had to administer myself in the form of a daily injection. The drug treatment then continued for about two weeks. After my natural cycle has then been suppressed, I was given a type of fertility hormone known as a gonadotrophin. I had to take this as a daily injection for around 12 days to help increase the number of eggs I produced. As the drug treatment happened, the clinic monitored my progress through vaginal ultrasound scans and blood tests. During this treatment phase there was a chance my body could suffer side effects such as hot flushes, feeling down or irritable, headaches, restlessness, and ovarian hyper stimulation syndrome (OHSS), which is the most serious side effect as this can cause symptoms such as a swollen stomach, stomach pains, nausea and vomiting. When I was told about the side effects, I again asked myself, Why me?

The last thing I needed was to suffer these awful side effects and then to be told the treatment had been unsuccessful. It was touch and go as to whether my body was going to ever produce any eggs, however I had to stay positive and hold onto that 1% chance because if I didn't try, I would always have been wondering what if?

For the first few days Dave had to do my injections for me as I was too scared. The problem was he was going away after a few days so I had to learn how to do them myself. Luckily, my friend showed me a cool trick were you have to touch your belly with the point of the needle and see if you can feel anything. If you can, that means there is muscle underneath. (However, in my case it was probably more like fat!) Then, if you find an area that doesn't hurt when you touch, this indicates it as a perfect area — free of muscle, which means the needle goes in much easier and without any pain. After a few days I put the technique into action and, from then on, I administered the drugs myself.

> **TOP TIP FOR INJECTING YOURSELF**
> Touch your belly with the point of the needle. If you can feel the sharp scratch, it indicates there is muscle underneath. Keep moving the needle until you find an area where you can't feel anything. This area is free of muscle, making it less painful and doesn't cause discomfort or bruise the skin.

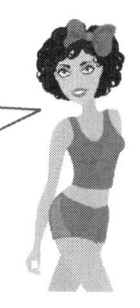

Amongst all of this, the time had come for Dave to go and give his semen specimen sample. Dave was horrified by the whole idea of turning up to the clinic knowing that everyone there knew what he was going to be doing. I don't think I have ever seen Dave looking so uncomfortable — and that was just when he was talking about it, never mind doing it! Dave was required to produce a semen sample on the day of egg collection and was advised to abstain for 2-3 days prior to producing his sample. If the period of abstinence is more than 7-10 days, the quality of the semen sample may become poor. Due to Dave's departure to lead a group of people up Kilimanjaro and his return being planned for the day of collection, this meant he would have to do his sample before he left. In an ideal world they like the sperm sample to be fresh and done on the day it is needed to fertilize the eggs for optimum results. (Of course, you will have read a bit about how Dave felt about all this back in Chapter Eight.)

One week into treatment and the odds were not looking good; my body wasn't producing as many eggs as they were hoping for so they considered whether or not treatment should carry on. Dave and I were not prepared to give up easily and decided we wanted carry on with treatment. We are so glad that we did because, although my body only managed to produce three eggs, this meant that, with the four I already had, I now had seven eggs.

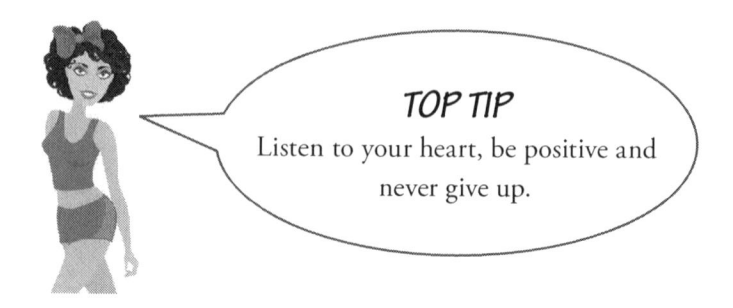

> **TOP TIP**
> Listen to your heart, be positive and never give up.

Ideally they like you to have 10 eggs as this gives you a higher chance of retrieving enough to fertilise. They say if you have 10 eggs to begin with, you will probably only retrieve 7, with only 2 or 3 from that 7 surviving the fertilisation process. This is why our chances of coming away with any embryos would be a miracle.

A date was arranged for the collection of my eggs but, before this could happen, they had to give me a hormone injection 38 hours prior to mature the eggs.

Wednesday, 21st October 2014 – Egg Collection Day

It is the day of egg collection. But this is no Easter Sunday running around to find little foil-covered chocolates hiding behind trees! Dave is away and I've had a stressful journey, arriving late so my time slot was delayed. On the way to the ward, which seemed as though they were taking me to a basement, the corridor felt very cold. There is some building work going on and when we got to the end of the corridor there was this rickety old lift that came crashing down. The doors squeaked open and I wondered whether I would make it to the first floor! When I arrived at the ward the doctors and nurses were rushing around ready to prep me. There were a few forms to go through and sign; as we were going through them the anaesthetist noticed I was chewing gum – she was not happy! She asked in a very stern tone, "Did you not read the instructions?" But I hadn't received any information by post; it was given verbally and I remember being told no food or drink. I didn't realise that meant NO chewing gum! My heart sank as my slot now had to be put back by two hours. On the bright side, I utilised my time by writing about my egg collection experience so far in this diary!

TOP TIP
Chewing gum is food! When you are told no food or drink before a procedure, that includes chewing gum!

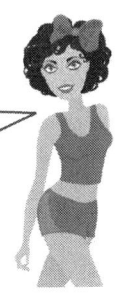

The Shock Factor

Two hours later I was given a gown and a sexy pair of surgical stockings to wear. When we arrived at the operating theatre there were quite a few doctors and nurses, as well as the anaesthetist. I started to feel very nervous, even more so with there being so many people in the room. They positioned me on the bed and connected me to the machine ready for sedation. The fear gripped me as I had no idea what to expect, apart from that I was only going to be sedated and not put to sleep. This freaked me out a little bit because I kept thinking, 'What if I can see everyone gathered round looking at my lady garden?' The sedation started as I was asked to put my legs in the stirrups. It felt so undignified!

Whilst sedated, my eggs were going to be collected using ultrasound guidance. This is a hollow needle attached to an ultrasound probe and is used to collect the eggs from the follicles on each ovary. Thankfully I had no idea what was happening and couldn't feel anything.

All in all, despite the slight humiliation of the position, it wasn't really that bad. I felt minimal pain, just like period pains. After the collection you can experience some cramps, feel a little sore and bruised and/or experience a small amount of bleeding — a bit like when you have your menstrual cycle.

Back at the ward I was told they had managed to retrieve three eggs out of the seven. I was so happy and, although I knew they still had to survive the fertilisation process, I stayed positive and was very hopeful. Given that two weeks previously we had been told the chance of IVF actually working was very low, the fact that we now had three eggs was fantastic!

As I was resting and feeling content, knowing that what I had just been through was definitely worth it, Dave arrived. This meant he could give a fresh sample. (There was one benefit to my chewing gum scenario in that this allowed him more time to get to the hospital, even though this was not the method in my madness — but they do say things happen for a reason!) His poor feet didn't even touch the hospital floor before they were carting him off for a fresh specimen, still in his hiking clothes and boots.

Not only had he just spent six days taking a group up one of the highest freestanding mountains, Kilimanjaro, he had also raced back from Heathrow airport and it had taken him five hours to get to me. We both knew that having a fresh sample would give us a better chance and, surely after having just climbed Kilimanjaro, those little tadpoles must be feeling stronger (maybe they were still in their hiking clothes and boots).

Dave came back looking flustered but with a look of relief on his face — only to be expected I suppose! We sat for the next hour chatting and laughing about the whole IVF experience and sharing our stories about his latest adventure and my medical escapades.

It would be a couple of days before we knew whether the fertilisation process had been a success.

> *Friday, 23rd November 2014 – Receiving the news*
>
> *Although I couldn't wait to find out whether the fertilisation procedure had been successful, a part of me was scared in case it was not the result I was hoping for. I couldn't cope with being told everything I had gone through had been for nothing and I would never be able to conceive any more children on top of everything else. I picked up the phone to hear Dr Fitzgerald at the other end. 'Hello Sarah, I'm phoning to give you the good news; two of the embryos have survived the fertilisation process.' I went silent as I absorbed the wonderful news. My belly did summersaults with the excitement.*
>
> *I couldn't wait to get off the phone to tell Dave. Everything we had been through now seems worthwhile. We are so thankful that we followed our hearts and listened to our gut instinct.*

We don't know whether or not I will still be able to conceive naturally, but we now have the comfort of knowing that we have two frozen embryos patiently waiting for when the time is right.

CHAPTER ELEVEN

One Year On

It's been 12 months since finishing treatment and everything is moving in the right direction. There have been many moments of change and plenty of emotions (tears, lots of tears). I often felt scared during treatment, but especially since finishing treatment. I hit a real low as the realisation of what I had been through hit me harder that I thought it would. It was a bit like being left to find the last remaining pieces of the jigsaw and having to figure out where it fits in the puzzle. Suddenly, after months of appointments and advice, I felt I was left to deal with the aftermath on my own, to return to the 'normal' life I had before cancer dealt its devastating blow. I found it challenging, as the life I knew before was not the life I was living now; it was a 'new' normal. I had to try to find a way of adapting to fit in. I quickly realised that life was never going to be like it was before and began to learn how to live my life after cancer.

When I was diagnosed I had never anticipated the journey being as intense and emotional as it has been. I have dealt with my situation better than I would have ever thought possible but at times struggle with coming to terms with what has just happened. My body and mind have slowly started to absorb the magnitude of what it has just been through and, to an extent, I am now suffering with post-traumatic stress.

It has been very difficult getting my head that just over 12 months ago I was like any normal 32-year-old, living a normal, happy life. All of a sudden I was hit with the devastating news that I had breast cancer; not only did I have to deal with the fact I had breast cancer, I had to come to terms with the fact that it was a stage 3 cancer, which meant it was very aggressive. In such a short space of time I had to accept that I would have to go through chemotherapy treatment and have a mastectomy. How does this happen? How can you go from being perfectly healthy to, within a couple of hours, your whole world being turned upside down and your life in turmoil. Having to get my head around the fact that I was about to embark on a horrific journey with operations and chemotherapy was the biggest challenge. It left me terrified and fighting for my life.

I still remember the moment so vividly like it was only yesterday, when Dave and I were sat in the hospital waiting anxiously for the results. It was a beautiful sunny day with clear blue skies. I knew that after that day, life was going to change in some way. I had already made the decision that if the biopsy results were negative but the genetic testing results confirmed that I was a BRCA carrier, and then I was going to have a double mastectomy to reduce my risks in the future. However, nothing prepared me for what I was about to hear. It felt like I had been kicked in the stomach and all of a sudden my life had turned into a life of uncertainty. It felt dark and I felt fearful of my future. Knowing I had to have chemo was the most horrific part, as I knew the extent of the side effects. At some point I would lose my beautiful long hair, which I had had since I was a little girl. However I also knew that chemo was the most important part of the treatment plan as it was my only lifeline — losing my hair seemed insignificant compared with losing my life. On the way home, Dave and I didn't speak; we were both in stunned silence as the seriousness of my diagnosis started to sink in. We then had to decide how we were going to tell our beautiful daughter, who was only four-years-old, that her mummy was poorly. As soon as I saw Lillie, my fear turned into strength as I realised that dying was not an option. I was going to do everything I needed to do in order to get myself better so I could be there to watch her grow up.

In some ways, my journey is over but, in another way, it has only just begun. Twelve months on I'm still here and have kicked cancer's arse! However, it's not been an easy year; there have been many dark and challenging moments with times of loneliness and vulnerability, but there have also been times of fun and laughter. There have been so many positives from my journey, all of which have had a huge impact on my life. I have come to realise how powerful your mindset is and that I have more strength than I ever thought possible.

Now I am embracing the new me! Making the decision to write this book was a big step on my journey. I hope it inspires you and other men or women who may be on their own journey now or may have to face a similar situation in the future, whether or not it is you who has been diagnosed with cancer or a friend or member of your family. My breast cancer page has has been more successful than I ever could have imagined. I also set up a private support group, called the 'Butterfly Breast Cancer Group', and organise themed events each month to bring women together to support each other, socialise and have fun in beautiful locations. Visit my website, *www.sarahsstory.co.uk*, for dates and information on forthcoming events.

As much as I wish I hadn't experienced this and will never forget what I have been through (and I have the scars to prove it), it has now become part of my life…but now in a positive way. It has created lots of fantastic opportunities to help and inspire others and to bring women together to share stories and support each other. I have met so many beautiful and inspirational ladies along the way who will be lifelong friends and I am looking forward to meeting lots more in the future. There are so many exciting ventures coming up in the future, so watch this space!

AFTERWORD

I never imagined this would be how my book would end; however I couldn't have wished for a happier ending. After everything we have been through, including IVF and against all odds, on Thursday 20th October 2016, I found out we are expecting our second baby, which is a complete surprise and an absolute miracle! Receiving the news has made everything worthwhile and makes you realise that there is hope after having cancer.

I'm even more enthusiastic to see what the future holds and where my journey will now lead. We are so excited and looking forward to the arrival of our new baby in summer 2017.

To be continued…

ABOUT SARAH

Sarah is 34, married to Dave and mother to her beautiful daughter, Lillie. On the 22nd of September 2014, her life changed when she was diagnosed with breast cancer. Although plunged into a strange and surreal dream, once she had absorbed the devastating news, she knew she was going to take control of the situation before it took control of her. From the start, Sarah was determined to approach the future in a positive way and use her journey to help others on a similar path or those who may find themselves in a similar situation in the future. She decided to write a book about her experiences, to share the high and lows, and the lessons learned throughout in the hope that she can help and inspire others undergoing their own battle with cancer.

Following her diagnosis, Sarah set up a Facebook page called Sarah's story — beating breast cancer one day at a time, where she shares each step of her journey. She also established the 'Butterfly cancer networking group' on Facebook, so that women going through cancer can chat to other women going through similar experiences and offer each other support and advice. Sarah now organises themed events every couple of months, which bring women together to socialise and have fun whilst raising money for cancer charities.

Sarah now shares her story by speaking at events and on the radio and raising awareness in the media. The rest of the time she enjoys time with her family, including Timmy the rabbit and Daisy, Maisy, Milly and Tilly the chickens. She is also the founder of Lilia's Beauty School, which keeps her very busy.

ST LUKE'S HOSPICE

St Luke's care for adults living in central and southern Cheshire who are suffering from cancer and other life limiting illnesses, serving a population of around 280,000. The Hospice opened in 1988 thanks to the incredible foresight of and donations received from the local community. 28 years later they continue to offer 24 hour care to local people, as well as their services offered in Day Hospice, out-patient clinics, complementary therapies, bereavement support and many other services.

They are often called a small hospice with a big heart because they passionately want to make a difference to the quality of people's lives; enabling them to live rather than exist. They are trusted by people when they are at their most vulnerable. Each year they support around 1,000 local adults and children through their varied services and constantly look to develop new services as the needs of the community change.

Today, donations mean more than ever; they are a charity which means all our services are provided free of charge, so over 80% of their running costs come from donations. For every £1 you give 80p goes directly to patient care, and the remaining 20p helps them to raise another £1. Every penny you give will make a difference. Thank you.

To donate to St Luke's Hospice visit
stlukes-hospice.co.uk/ways-to-support-us/donate/donate

* * * *

MACMILLAN

When you have cancer, you don't just worry about what will happen to your body, you worry about what will happen to your life. Whether it's concerns about who you can talk to, planning for the extra costs or what to do about work, at Macmillan they understand how a cancer diagnosis can affect everything.

No one should face cancer alone. So when you need someone to turn to, Macmillan are here. Right from the moment you're diagnosed, through your treatment and beyond, they are a constant source of support, giving you the energy and inspiration to help you take back control of your life.

For support, information or if you just want to chat, call Macmillan free on **0808 808 00 00** (Monday to Friday, 9am–8pm) or visit **macmillan.org**

USEFUL WEBSITES

St Luke's Hospice
stlukes-hospice.co.uk

Macmillan
macmillan.org.uk

Navitas Holistic Therapy & Reiki Centre
navitascentre.co.uk

Toni Mackenzie
innerdepths.co.uk

Chris McDermott
reconstellation.com

Tonje Olsen (Physiotherapist)
tonje_olsen_87@hotmail.com

Carol Roberts (Personal Trainer)
carolroberts1974@hotmail.co.uk

Kate Marshall (Yoga and Reiki)
inspiringenergy.co.uk

Didis Boutique (vintage dresses)
lovedidis.co.uk

Gayna Cooper (sells a range of natural products that contain no nasties)
tropicskincare.co.uk/shop/gaynacooper

Drain Dollies (surgical drain bags)
draindollies.co.uk

Bravissimo (lingerie and clothing)
bravissimo.com and bravissimo.com/pepperberry

Edge Travel Worldwide (setting exciting goals which enhance quality of life, give hope and provide life changing experiences)
edgetravelworldwide.com

Made in the USA
Columbia, SC
01 May 2017